W9-BJJ-268

Date Due

AUG 31 1995

M.R.P. HALL

W.J. MacLENNAN

M.D.W. LYE

Medical Care of the Elderly

THIRD EDITION

JOHN WILEY & SONS

Chichester · New York · Brisbane · Toronto · Singapore

Copyright © 1993 by John Wiley & Sons Ltd,
Baffins Lane, Chichester,
West Sussex PO19 1UD, England

Other Wiley Editorial Offices

John Wiley & Sons, Inc., 605 Third Avenue,
New York, NY 10158–0012, USA

Jacaranda Wiley Ltd, G.P.O. Box 859, Brisbane,
Queensland 4001, Australia

John Wiley & Sons (Canada) Ltd, 22 Worcester Road,
Rexdale, Ontario M9W 1L1, Canada

John Wiley & Sons (SEA) Pte Ltd, 37 Jalan Pemimpin #05-04,
Block B, Union Industrial Building, Singapore 2057

Library of Congress Cataloging-in-Publication Data
Hall, Michael R. P.
    Medical care of the elderly / M.R.P. Hall, W.J. MacLennan, M.D.W.
Lye.—3rd ed.
       p.   cm.
    Includes bibliographical references and index.
    ISBN 0 471 93997 8
    1. Geriatrics.   2. Aged—Medical care.   I. MacLennan, W. J.
II. Lye, M. D. W.   III. Title.
    [DNLM: 1. Aged.   2. Geriatrics.   3. Health Services for the Aged—
case studies.   WT 30 H178m 1993]
    RC952.H245 1993
    362.1'9897—dc20
    DNLM/DLC
    for Library of Congress   93-13619
                                                                    CIP

British Library Cataloguing in Publication Data

A catalogue record for this book is available from the British Library

ISBN 0 471 93997 8

Typeset in 11/13pt Photina by Photo·graphics, Honiton, Devon
Printed and bound in Great Britain by Biddles Ltd, Guildford, Surrey

CONTENTS

AUTHORS' ADDRESSES

M.R.P. Hall BM BCh FRCP FRCPE
Professor Emeritus of Geriatric Medicine
The University,
Southampton SO9 5NH

W.J. MacLennan MD FRCP (Lond., Ed. & Glasg.)
Professor of Geriatric Medicine
University of Edinburgh, City Hospital,
Greenbank Drive, Edinburgh EH10 5SB

M.D.W. Lye MD FRCP
Professor of Geriatric Medicine
Royal Liverpool University Hospital,
Prescot Street, PO Box 147,
Liverpool L69 3BX

PREFACE

Again seven years have passed since the last edition of this book. The numbers of people in the older age groups—those over 75, 80 and 85 years—have increased as predicted and forecasts suggest that this trend will continue. Indeed, the total number aged over 65 years will increase to over 12 million in the course of the next 30 to 40 years. We do not view this demographic advance as a crisis, timebomb or catastrophe but rather a measure of past success and a future challenge.

Moreover, it is not the continuing increase in the numbers of elderly that has been the stimulus for another edition. The reason has been twofold. Firstly, the last seven years have seen the development of many technical advances in medical science that have been and are of great benefit to the medical care of the elderly. In the previous edition we resisted the temptation to include all new advances in knowledge in each field. Some of these advances are now current practice and must be included in a new edition. Consequently, we have reviewed the total content, and many of the chapters have been completely rewritten to incorporate new material. Secondly, the NHS and the Community Health Act 1990 is now law and becomes operative this year. As far as is possible this has been taken into account and the new role of the local authority described in Chapter 4. This, together with the demographic changes, means that more people will be involved in the overall care of the elderly. If a good "seamless service" is to be provided, then wider appreciation of the application of medical care will be necessary.

We have retained the original form of the book, but have provided 10 new case histories to reflect the type of patient being seen in two professorial units. We have continued to emphasise the team approach, for our book was originally intended as a guide for the team and this intention remains. Indeed, now that one of us has joined the "geriatriclog" (cf. "banderlog" in Kipling's *Jungle*

Book), the need for an integrated approach to the potential patient has assumed an even greater importance!

While this book is primarily a medical handbook, which has been written from a hospital perspective, we believe that it will also be of value to *all* those working in the community and not only those doctors who are taking Diplomas of Geriatric Medicine. Nurses have always undertaken a major role in the care of the elderly, and this will increase. Nurse training has altered and we believe that this book will be as valuable to the undergraduate nurse as it will be to those already qualified, as well as remedial therapists, social workers and others who work in this interesting field of health care.

As in the previous editions we have tried to link the cases as closely as possible to the text of the chapters and vice versa. We hope that by referring "back and forth" readers will obtain a greater insight into the care of elderly patients which will help them to continue to meet the challenges of this fascinating and rewarding subject.

January 1993

M.R.P. Hall
W.J. MacLennan
M.D.W. Lye

CASE HISTORIES AND COMMENTARY

CASE 1: MALE, AGED 76 YEARS

History

This patient was referred to the geriatric service because of failure to mobilise after surgery for a bleeding duodenal ulcer. He had been admitted 6 weeks earlier with an acute haematemesis followed by melaena. There was a vague history that 4 years previously he had been prescribed ranitidine for post-prandial discomfort but this had been stopped after approximately 6 months' treatment. His only other problem was long-standing painful arthritis of the right knee for which he took various medicines which he bought over the counter (OTC) from the chemist (OTC medicines).

At the time of his admission the surgeons were reluctant to operate because of his poor "general condition and confusion" (see Chapter 9). He was transfused 3 units of blood and the duodenal ulcer treated by laser bicap diathermy. Unfortunately he bled again, became hypotensive and was transfused a further 7 units of blood before undergoing emergency surgery where a bleeding vessel was tied and a pyloroplasty and vagotomy successfully performed. He was managed postoperatively on the intensive therapy unit (ITU) where with the help of a ventilator, antibiotics and a "renal" dopamine regimen he recovered from bilateral bronchopneumonia. His conscious level was low and it was concluded that he had suffered a stroke when hypotensive. He returned to the general surgical ward after 3 days but in spite of active encouragement by the nurses and intensive physiotherapy he failed to mobilise and was referred to the geriatric service.

Examination

The patient presented with a withdrawn apathetic depressed picture and was reluctant to mobilise. There was specific cognitive impairment on formal testing (AMT—see Table 9.3) and he was disorientated in time and space. He had a black painful right heel limiting weight bearing (Chapter 5, "Bed sores"). Physical examination revealed considerable weight loss, an osteoarthritic deformity of the right knee (Chapter 7) and obvious signs of Parkinsonism or Parkinson's disease (Chapter 8). Formal testing (Hamilton Rating Scale) did not confirm a depressive illness. The hypokinesia of Parkinson's disease mimics a depressive illness and vice versa. Formal evaluation is mandatory (Chapter 6, "Depression").

Management

He was transferred to a geriatric rehabilitation ward where his nocturnal haloperidol was stopped. As there was little change in his Parkinsonian signs it was concluded that he was suffering from Parkinson's disease and not haloperidol-induced Parkinsonism. Paracetamol and a sheepskin heel cover were given for relief of pain and for protection respectively. It is impossible as well as dangerous to mobilise directly on damaged heels (Chapter 5, "Rehabilitation and the adjustment of the environment"). L-dopa with a high-dose decarboxylase inhibitor to prevent peripheral side effects (postural hypotension, gastric upset) was started and increased while his progress was monitored (timed walking distance, handwriting) by the physiotherapist. Subjective assessment of rehabilitation progress is mainly a waste of time. After 3 further weeks following a home visit it was apparent that the patient, who lived alone, would have to be completely independent as he obstinately refused all offers of help both formal and informal. After a full case conference, including the patient, a rehabilitation plan was agreed by all (Chapter 5, "The case conference"). He was referred for further occupational therapy and after a further 2 weeks was ready for discharge. Unfortunately he could not return home because the Gas Board had turned off the gas to his flat following a suspected leak. Potentially this could have been a disaster by demoralising and demotivating the patient and thus increasing his dependency. After 3 further weeks the gas was re-connected and the patient discharged with day hospital follow-up.

CASE 2: FEMALE, AGED 83 YEARS

History

The general practitioner contacted the registrar on call for the care of the elderly unit to report that the patient had become extremely muddled over the last 3 days, and that she had taken to her bed and become immobile.

She suffered from senile macular degeneration (Chapter 6) and had been registered blind for 4 years. She had severe deafness, and although she had been issued with a hearing aid, there had been difficulty in persuading her to use this. Hypertension had been diagnosed six years previously, and she was currently on nifedipine in a dose of 10 mg twice daily. She was also on digoxin in a dose of 62.5 μg daily. It was unclear why this had been started 3 years previously.

She was a widow who lived alone in a second floor tenement flat, and had been housebound for 6 years. A home help and a community nurse were in attendance 5 days a week. Her general practitioner had been concerned about her nutritional state for some time, and had been prescribing Feospan in a dose of 150 mg daily and one vitamin capsule daily.

Examination

She was admitted to the assessment unit the same day. On admission she was found to be cooperative, but she was confused, and unable to give a clear history. Although she was extremely deaf (Chapter 6), it was possible to administer a mental status questionnaire (Chapter 9) by using an electronic communicator. Her score was only 3/10.

Her tongue was dry, her eyes sunken and her skin lax and inelastic, but she had a trace of oedema of both ankles (Chapter 10). There was little body fat, and there was generalised muscle wasting. Examination of her fundi revealed that there was patchy pigmentation affecting both maculae.

Her pulse was regular, was of good volume and had a rate of 90 beats/minute. She had a forceful apex beat which was displaced laterally and downwards. There were a few coarse crepitations at both lung bases, but these were more marked on the right side.

4

Case 1.

Problems	Effects	Actions
Duodenal ulcer	(i) Anaemia	(a) ?how long ?aspirin (GP)
	(ii) Acute bleed	(b) Urgent surgery (S)
	(iii) Nutritional deficit	(c) Check dietary intake (DT)
Acute illness	(i) Confusion	(a) Reassure (D, N)
		(b) Pain relief (D, N)
		(c) Do not sedate (D)
Postoperative dependency	(i) Hypostatic pneumonia	(a) Antibiotics (D)
	(ii) Deep vein thrombosis	(b) Mobilise (N, PT)
Heel pressure sore	(i) Immobility	(a) Prevent (N, PT)
		(b) Treat (N, PT)
Muscle wasting	(i) Immobility	(a) Prevent (N, PT)
		(b) Treat (N, PT)
Parkinson's disease	(i) Immobility	(a) Diagnosis (D, PG)
	(ii) "Apathy, depression"	(b) L-dopa drugs (D)
	(iii) Dietary intake	(c) Re-enable (PT, OT, DT, N)
Discharge delay	(i) Demoralisation	(a) Gas Board (SW, D)
Lives alone		(b) Day hospital follow-up (D. N. SW)

Key: D = doctor; N = nurse; PT = physiotherapist; PG = psychogeriatrician; OT = occupational therapist; SW = social worker; S = surgeon; GP = general practitioners; DT = dietitian.

Although there were no abnormal neurological signs she was unable to stand without the support of two people.

Management

A chest X-ray revealed that there was mild pulmonary congestion associated with increased pulmonary vascular markings. In addition, there was evidence of a patchy consolidation at the right lower zone. Since it proved impossible to obtain a specimen of sputum, it was decided to treat the bronchopneumonia empirically with amoxycillin in an oral dose of 250 mg three times daily.

Biochemical analysis of a sample of blood revealed that her serum sodium, chloride and potassium concentrations were within normal limits, but that her blood urea concentration was elevated to 20.8 mmol/l. In view of the fact that she also had evidence of cardiac failure, it was decided not to give her parenteral fluids but to push these orally. On this regimen, there was a progressive fall in her blood urea concentration.

Management of her congestive cardiac failure presented problems. Because she had an elevated blood urea concentration, it was decided not to prescribe a diuretic. Treatment was withheld until her blood urea had returned to normal. At this stage, she still had some ankle oedema, and there were a few coarse crepitations at her lung bases. She was given a test dose of 6.25 mg of captopril (Chapter 10). This did not induce severe hypotension, and she was started on enalapril in a dose of 5 mg daily. Since she did not have atrial fibrillation, it was unlikely that digoxin was contributing to control of her cardiac failure, and it was discontinued.

Nifedipine was discontinued before the angiotensin-converting enzyme (ACE) inhibitor was started. The blood pressure did not fall below 160/95 mmHg even when the dose of enalapril was increased to 10 mg daily. It was felt that more aggressive treatment was not indicated in a woman of her age with mental impairment and multiple pathology.

She was rather agitated over the first few hours of admission. This was managed by caring for her in a quiet room, and providing her with frequent reassurance (Chapter 9). Sedation was unnecessary, and her confusion settled with resolution of her chest infection, and control of the dehydration. The score on a mental status questionnaire repeated at this stage was 7/10.

The senile macular degeneration had already been reviewed by an ophthalmologist. Both eyes had been affected when she was assessed initially so that active treatment was inappropriate. However, she had derived considerable benefit from being registered blind.

She was visited by a hearing therapist (Chapter 6) who counselled her and trained her in the use of a hearing aid.

The physiotherapist arranged walking exercises and, after one week, she was walking with support from a tripod and was able to transfer without help. She was able to dress if her clothes were placed on a chair close to her. A kitchen assessment was less successful in that she had difficulty in finding her way round the unit, on account of her poor vision, but she was much more competent in her own kitchen.

There was concern that she had neglected her nutritional status in the past. Meals were organised at a day centre twice per week, and meals-on-wheels sent to her on the other 5 days. Support from a home help and community nurse was continued.

The advantages of admission to residential care were reviewed. She was isolated in a second floor flat, and was at risk from self-neglect and injury. Conversely she valued her privacy and independence, and it was agreed, therefore, that continued support in her own home was the most appropriate action.

CASE 3: MALE, AGED 68 YEARS

History

This man was brought by his wife to the accident and emergency department having sustained a 3–4 tonic–clonic seizure. He had served in the merchant navy for many years and had suffered an acute stroke leading to a dense right hemiplegia, 4 years previously. In the past, when investigated at a neurological institute, he had been found to have positive serology for syphilis. In spite of intensive penicillin therapy there had been no change in his hemiplegia. His wife's serology was negative. After a computed tomographic (CT) scan he had been told that he had had a vascular stroke, that he should stop smoking and that nothing more could be done. He was discharged and provided with a transit wheelchair. His wife, fortunately, a physically and mentally strong woman, had managed to look after him, since then, without help. She had not contacted his general practitioner during this period.

Case 2.

Problems	Effects	Actions
Bronchopneumonia	(i) Confusion (ii) Breathlessness	(a) Antibiotics (D) (b) Chest physiotherapy (PT)
Congestive cardiac failure	(i) Oedema (ii) Breathlessness	(a) ACE inhibitor (D)
Hypertension	(i) Stroke (ii) Cardiac failure (iii) Renal failure	(a) ACE inhibitor (D)
Dehydration	(i) High blood urea (ii) Confusion	(a) Push oral fluids (N)
Confusion (delirium)	(i) Mental distress (ii) Noisiness and disturbance (iii) Personal injury	(a) Treat underlying cause (D) (b) Quietness and reassurance (N) (c) Careful sedation (D)
Macular degeneration	(i) Blindness (ii) Falls (iii) Boredom (iv) Isolation (v) Problems with self-care and cooking	(a) Registration (O) (b) Home help (SW) (c) Talking book (L) (d) Visits (V) (e) Dressing training (OT) (f) Kitchen training (OT)
Deafness	(i) Isolation (ii) Mental disorder	(a) Hearing aid (A) (b) Counselling (H)
Poor nutrition	(i) Poor health	(a) Meals-on-wheels, Day centre (SW, DT)

Key: A = audiologist; D = doctor; DT = dietitian; H = hearing therapist; L = librarian; N = nurse; O = ophthalmologist; OT = occupational therapist; PT = physiotherapist; SW = social worker; V = volunteer.

The sudden onset of fitting frightened her but otherwise she was remarkably uncomplaining. Detailed questioning revealed that he had been incontinent of urine for the previous 2 years which she had managed with proprietary pads. For the same time he had been depressed, wishing to die and latterly had become paranoid about his wife. He had accused her of neglecting him and seeing other men while out shopping. This had led to physical aggression and on occasions she had not been able to avoid injury.

Examination

When his post-ictal drowsiness had resolved (after approximately 72 hours) he was found to be mentally alert though withdrawn and uncooperative. The elderly brain takes a long time to recover from electrical or metabolic insults (Chapter 9). Neurologically he had signs of a dense right hemiplegia with contractures of the arm and hand. Adequate rehabilitation at the time of his initial stroke could possibly have prevented contractures thus making management by his wife easier (Chapter 8, "Completed stroke"). Identible faeces were palpable through the anterior abdominal wall and on rectal examination. Lack of mobility is a potent cause of constipation and faecal impaction and often leads to urinary incontinence (Chapter 14). His general fitness was good in spite of excessive cigarette smoking. The skin and pressure areas were intact— a tribute to his wife's hard work. Functionally, he needed two nurses to transfer him from bed to chair to commode. He was unable or unwilling to wash himself or assist with dressing. He was able to feed himself but was exceedingly messy. He was observed to periodically cough and splutter following drinks but not solids. Detailed monitoring by the night nurses confirmed early morning wakening and the Hamilton Rating Scale suggested a diagnosis of a depressive illness (Chapter 6, "Depression").

Management

Even though this was the first recorded fit, in view of his cerebrovascular damage he was prescribed sodium valproate. His wife confirmed that following his fit her husband's dependency had increased and that he was less able to help with transfers etc. The faecal impaction was treated with a series of enemas which, combined with regular toileting regime, kept him continent on the geriatric assessment ward. Laxative agents were prescribed but enemas continued to be required at approximately weekly intervals. Careful observation and monitoring are required to elaborate an appropriate regimen to manage constipation. An attempt was made to persuade him to take thickened drinks to prevent aspiration. He complained vehemently that "he was not drinking wallpaper paste" and his doctor had to agree with him. The speech therapist taught him swallowing routines to minimise aspiration which, commonly, is not always appreciated in patients with stroke especially in the acute stage (Chapter 8, "Assessment of impairment").

He was transferred to the geriatric rehabilitation ward with the objective of making him less dependent on his wife, so easing her strain, rather than more independent himself. The physiotherapist therefore spent most of her time working with both the patient and his wife, showing her lifting/transferring techniques (Chapter 5, "Rehabilitation and the adjustment of the environment"). She was a most willing pupil: he was not. A psychogeriatric assessment advised that formal antidepressants might be worth a trial. This combined with "counselling" by individuals from the whole multidisciplinary team may have improved his mood and cooperation; the improvement, however, was marginal. Attempts by nurses and occupational therapists to get him to help with self-care were resisted: "my wife does that for me so I am not going to bother". He was offered a single-drive wheelchair but refused to use it giving the same reason. In this situation it is vital that the rehabilitation team work together and support each other. In the face of an ungrateful, uncooperative and aggressive patient it is easy to "reject the patient" (Chapter 4, "Difficult personalities"). A home visit revealed that the patient's wife with the assistance of various relatives had made good use of informal adaptations, particularly in the downstairs bathroom and toilet. However, referral was made to the local social services department to provide a ramp to allow wheelchair access to the house. Because of the delay in implementing this, the patient's brother-in-law built it himself after the patient was discharged. The social worker had arranged transport to a local day centre on a weekly basis, but after a few visits he refused to attend. Regular respite admissions were offered but the wife was reluctant to accept. Often close carers will develop feelings of guilt if they accept offers of statutory help, etc. Sometimes, to circumvent this, it is helpful if medical staff make a recommendation "in the patient's interest". It was eventually agreed that if she gave 2 or 3 weeks' notice, respite admissions would be provided "on demand". Professionals have to recognise that the provision of care is best if operated on "a partnership of equals'" basis.

Over the next few months he was admitted at approximately 6 week intervals for never more than a week at a time. The ward nurses built up a good relationship with the wife and she told them that the aggressive outbursts had recurred. Later she was able to discuss them with the doctors who, having confirmed that they were not epileptic in nature, sedated him with haloperidol. Unfortunately initial doses were too high and he became totally immobile with hypotension and drowsiness (Chapter 5, "Drug therapy"). Over the ensuing months different dosages and different drugs were tried but with little benefit—too little, not effective—too much, effective, but physically more disabled. Eventually the wife announced that she knew when the aggression was going to start and what dose of haloperidol would be best for each occasion. She was given a free hand and was proved right. Knowledge of drug pharmacokinetics and pharmacodynamics cannot replace close and constant observation. She assumed responsibility for the institution, frequency of administration and dose of haloperidol.

CASE 4: FEMALE, AGED 82 YEARS

History

A geriatrician was asked to perform a domiciliary visit on a patient who had been having recurrent falls over the last 4 weeks. It was impossible to obtain a clear history from her, but the warden of the sheltered housing complex in which she lived stated that she had been extremely forgetful ever since she had moved there 2 years ago. Particular problems were that she frequently locked herself out of her flat, that her personal hygiene was poor, and that she dressed carelessly often appearing out of doors in her dressing gown and slippers. Over the last 4 weeks her home help had found her lying on the floor on at least four occasions. Despite the fact that there was an alarm system in the flat, the patient had not used this to summon help after an accident, possibly because she had difficulty in understanding how the system worked.

Case 3.

Problems	Effects	Actions
Fits	(i) Possible trauma (ii) Increased dependency (iii) Panic in wife	(a) Anti-epileptics (D) (b) Reassurance and explanation (N)
Faecal impaction	(i) Constipation (ii) Urinary incontinence	(a) Laxative (D) (b) Enemas and monitor (N, CN) (c) Laundry, social services (SW)
Immobility	(i) Dependency (ii) Pressure on wife	(a) Maximise function (PT) (b) Washing/dressing (OT)
Swallowing	(i) Aspiration (ii) Chest infection	(a) Alter dietary consistency (DT, C)
Depression	(i) Dependency	(a) Assessment, treatment (PG)
Aggression	(i) Abuse—patient or wife (ii) Carer breakdown	(a) Counselling (D, N, SW) (b) Haloperidol (D, wife)
Home support	(i) Carer breakdown	(a) Respite care (D) (b) Day centre (SW) (c) Home visit/adaptions (OT, SW)

Key: C = cook; CN = community nurse; D = doctor; DT = dietitian; N = nurse; OT = occupational therapist; PG = psychogeriatri-cian; PT = physiotherapist; SW = social worker.

Examination

The patient had a pleasant personality and a good social facade. Formal rating with a mental status questionnaire revealed that she scored only 2/10 (Chapter 9). Her conjunctivae were extremely pale and she had marked koilonychia. She had gross oedema of her left leg, and considerable tenderness in her left calf.

She was ataxic, and took small shuffling steps. Her face showed little expression and she did not swing her arms when she walked. Tone in all four limbs was normal, however, and she had no tremor.

Management

In view of the multiplicity of her problems, and the increasing difficulty she was experiencing in coping with her self-care it was decided to admit her to the geriatric assessment unit.

Consideration was given to the large number of factors which could have been responsible for her falls (Chapter 8, "Falls"). The most probable explanation was her ataxia and akinesia. In view of the fact that there was no rigidity or tremor, it was decided that the condition was unlikely to be due to Parkinson's disease, but that it was associated with senile dementia of Alzheimer type (SDAT). A course of walking exercises restored her confidence and improved her balance.

Analysis of a blood sample revealed that she had a haemoglobin of 9.7 g/dl, and that the erythrocytes were microcytic and hypochromic. The diagnosis was confirmed by a serum ferritin level of only 3 µg/l. Three samples of faeces were all positive when tested for blood.

Examination with a flexible sigmoidoscope revealed that there was extensive diverticular disease. A barium enema confirmed that the disease was confined to the descending and sigmoid colon, and that there were no abnormalities distal to this. The patient also was given a barium meal examination to check that there was only one pathology in the gastrointestinal tract. This was normal.

The anaemia was treated with ferrous sulphate in a dose of 200 mg three times daily, and the diverticular disease with mebeverine in a dose of 135 mg three times daily, and methylcellulose in a dose of 500 mg daily.

The unilateral leg oedema was diagnosed as a deep leg vein

thrombosis. Since the patient also had iron deficiency anaemia and gastrointestinal blood loss, treatment with anticoagulants was contraindicated. The oedema was managed by applying a one way stretch bandage from the foot to the groin.

When the erythrocyte sedimentation rate was checked as part of the routine investigation it was found to be 93 mm/1st hour. Serum immunoelectrophoresis revealed an increase in alpha-2 and gamma globulin but no other abnormalities, and chest X-ray was normal. Culture of a mid-stream specimen of urine identified a heavy growth of *Escherichia coli*. This was treated with amoxycillin in a dose of 250 mg three times daily (Chapter 13, "Renal and urinary tract infection").

Despite treatment of her anaemia and urinary tract infection, the mental test score remained unchanged. Evaluation by the occupational therapists established that she needed a great deal of guidance when dressing herself, and that she was extremely reluctant to wash. A medical social worker discussed the situation with the patient and her daughter, and it was decided that an appropriate option would be to seek a place in a nursing home. At this stage the nursing home liaison officer employed by the Health Board was contacted. After further evaluation of the needs of the patient, she made arrangements for her to visit a nursing home with a vacancy. The visit was a success, and the patient was admitted, with the fees being paid by social security supplementation. Over the next few weeks, the liaison officer visited on several occasions to ensure that the patient had settled in, and that both she and her daughter were happy with the arrangement.

CASE 5: FEMALE, AGED 98 YEARS

History

This frail elderly widow was referred by the orthopaedic surgeon because of failure to mobilise after hip replacement. The reason for her referral originally was stated to be that she had refused to consider giving up her totally inappropriate home and move into a nursing home. As far as the patient was concerned she was either going to go home or stay in hospital. The concerned consensus of the orthopaedic team, social workers and massed relatives was to no avail—she had lived in that area for more than 70 years, her husband had died in her present house and she was adamant that

Case 4.

Problems	Effects	Actions
Falls	(i) Trauma (ii) Hypothermia (iii) Loss of confidence (iv) Anxious relatives	(a) Diagnose cause (D) (b) Walking exercises (PT) (c) Walking aid (PT) (d) Safe environment (HV) (e) Sheltered housing (HD) (f) Personal alarm (SW)
Iron deficiency anaemia	(i) Symptoms, e.g. lethargy, breathlessness and dizziness	(a) Prescribe iron (D) (b) Blood transfusion (D) (c) Identify cause (D)
Diverticular disease	(i) Blood loss, anaemia (ii) Diarrhoea and pain	(a) Anticholinergic (D) (b) Increase "roughage" (DT) (c) Colonic resection (S)
Deep leg vein thrombosis	(i) Pulmonary embolism (ii) Leg oedema	(a) Anticoagulate (D) (b) Compression bandage (N) (c) Find and treat cause (D)
Urinary infection	(i) Frequency, dysuria and incontinence (ii) Confusion (iii) Septicaemia	(a) Obtain clean urine specimen for culture (N) (b) Antibiotic (D) (c) Identify cause (D)
Dementia	(i) Inability to manage activities of daily living (ii) Abnormal behaviour	(a) Assess ability (PG, OT) (b) Supported environment and health back-up (CPN, SW) (c) Institutional care (SW, LO)

Key: CPN = community psychiatric nurse; D = doctor; DT = dietitian; HD = housing department; HV = health visitor; LO = nursing home liaison officer; PG = psychogeriatrician; PT = physiotherapist; S = surgeon; SW = social worker.

she would do the same. She was the mother of 13 children of whom 8 were still living and had lived on her own in the large family home since her husband had died some 30 years ago. She was fiercely independent and indeed many called her cantankerous. She had been remarkably fit until approximately 2 years before her admission to the orthopaedic surgeons.

At that time she had become subject to recurrent falls (Chapter 8, "Falls"). She described the sequence of events as "coming over funny", light-headed and dizzy but not vertiginous. She did not lose consciousness and could initially abort an attack by sitting down. At first these attacks were occasional but latterly had become more frequent and more severe. She had been brought by her relatives to the accident and emergency department on two occasions in the previous year. After extensive X-rays, on both occasions, no bony injuries had been seen and she had been sent home with a referral to the social work department. Because of increased frequency of falling she became more reliant on her family and ceased leaving her house. Her final fall had occurred while getting out of bed and had caused her to fracture her femur. Unfortunately, because of ignorance, prejudice or ageism, old people have to "earn" their admission to hospital by fracturing bones! Most old ladies with recurrent falls have visited their local accident and emergency department three or four times over the preceding year. If junior doctors would subtract 40 years off the patient's age and treat accordingly, the aetiology of the recurrent falling (which is never due to age alone) would be diagnosed and treated before devastating complications arise.

Examination

When seen on the orthopaedic ward she was obviously dispirited if not clinically depressed. There was good pain-free movement of the hip and all other joints were satisfactory. There was some muscle wasting, particularly of the upper leg. There was pitting oedema of the ankles and a few scattered basal crepitations in the lungs. The pulse was 46 beats per minute with a good blood pressure. When asked to stand both arms were offered for lifting—a sure sign of induced (nurse/carer) dependency. When helped she was "backward leaning" and terrified of falling. Walking was impossible as her legs were thrust forward like sparrows' feet.

Management

She was transferred to the geriatric rehabilitation unit. A suspicion of hypothyroidism was not confirmed by thyroid function tests (Chapter 3, "Thyroid disease"). Mild heart failure (Chapter 10) was confirmed when a chest X-ray showed moderate cardiomegaly and some upper lobe venous distension. She was prescribed a diuretic with little effect. Standard ECG demonstrated sinus bradycardia and myocardial ischaemia. There was no postural drop in blood pressure on standing and no heart rate increase with limited exercise. This suggested that peripheral vascular resistance could be increased appropriately but chronological response of the heart was impaired. A 24 hour ECG confirmed overall sinus bradycardia with several episodes of sinus arrest—maximum duration 11 seconds (Chapter 10, "Cardiac arrhythmias"). Throughout this recording the patient was asymptomatic. The temporal relationship of arrhythmias to symptoms during 24 hour monitoring is very loose so a therapeutic trial of pacing or anti-arrhythmic drugs is usually warranted. Following insertion of an atrial demand pacemaker the patient's mood improved considerably though her physical capabilities did not change.

Much time was spent by doctors, nurses and social workers trying to assure her that the objective was to rehabilitate her so that she could return to her own home with appropriate support if necessary. Unfortunately the staff of the orthopaedic ward had colluded with her relatives and had produced a very negative prognosis based on inadequate information and assessment. Her extreme old age had overly impressed her carers. The nature of her "funny turns" was explained to her and her family. The physiotherapist used head-up tilt on a table to retrain her postural and positional reflexes (mechanoreceptors). Immobility from any cause, however brief, in ill old people leads to a vicious downward spiral of decreased reflex activity and decreasing mobility (Chapter 7, "Muscles"). When the physiotherapy took effect, after about 2 weeks, the first faltering steps with the physiotherapist rapidly improved to walking with one nurse. Human physical support was gradually reduced as her confidence improved. A major complication of repeated falls is extreme loss of confidence or outright fear. With the occupational therapist's help she rapidly became independent in dressing and self-care though she remained a liability in the hospital occupational therapy kitchen. Elderly patients rarely have high-tech kitchens in their homes!

Her home visit was arranged and it was only then that the hospital staff were confronted by the combined force of relatives' opposition (Chapter 4, "Relatives, friends and neighbours"). They were adamant that she could not live alone and they were unable and unwilling to provide continuous support especially at night. This was in spite of the fact that she probably did not need this! Most of the closest relatives were themselves quite elderly. The patient was persuaded that she would be happier and less of a burden on the rest of the family if she agreed to go into a home. The hospital social worker, even with the help of the patient's general practitioner, was unable to change the outcome and she was discharged to residential accommodation 9 weeks after first entering hospital (Chapter 4, "Residential accommodation"). Professionals have to accept that patients and/or their relatives must be free to make "wrong decisions". The patient's autonomy is paramount. The professionals should confine themselves to explaining all available options. In the vast majority of cases relatives should not take decisions for elderly patients. Such decisions would not be legally nor morally valid. Once the patient has made a decision the staff's responsibility is to support that decision however disappointing it may seem to them.

CASE 6: FEMALE, AGED 69 YEARS

History

After discussion of the patient with a registrar in the Care of the Elderly Unit her general practitioner sent her to the geriatric day hospital. Over the past 3 weeks she had had four "blackouts". Witnesses had told her that these had lasted about 15 minutes. They had not reported any abnormal movements during them. The patient was unaware of any prodromal symptoms. She had experienced similar attacks about 20 years ago, but these had eventually settled without treatment.

Over the last few months she had been troubled by pain in her lower back radiating down the back of her left leg. This had been investigated by an orthopaedic surgeon who had a particular interest in spinal lesions, and he had diagnosed this as sciatica associated with osteoarthritis. Over a much longer period of time she had been troubled by pain in her neck. This did not radiate into her

Case 5.

Problems	Effects	Actions
Extreme old age	(i) Frailty (ii) Elitism	(a) At risk (GP) (b) Nil
Sick sinus syndrome	Falls: (i) Fracture (ii) Loss of confidence (iii) Immobility (iv) Dependency (v) Arrhythmia	(a) Operation (S) (b) Re-mobilise (N, PT) (c) Exercise (PT, N) (d) Re-enable (OT, SW) (e) Pacemaker (D)
Cardiac failure	(i) Immobility	(a) Diuretics (D)
Family's anxiety	(i) Institutional care	(a) List options (D, N, SW) (b) Preserve patient's autonomy (all—professionals and family)

Key: D = doctor; GP = general practitioner; N = nurse; OT = occupational therapist; PT = physiotherapist; S = surgeon; SW = social worker.

upper limbs, and detailed questioning failed to elicit a relationship between neck movements and her blackouts.

Hypothyroidism (Chapter 13) had been identified 7 years previously and she was taking currently 75 μg of thyroxine daily.

Examination

The patient was alert and cooperative. She walked with a slight limp, but there was no evidence of Rombergism. There was painful limitation of neck movement, but this was not associated with any neurological symptoms. Movement of her lower spine was limited, and she resisted elevation of her straightened left leg to beyond 60 degrees.

There were no signs of Parkinsonism, corticospinal tract disease or cerebellar dysfunction. Her pulse was regular, there were no heart murmurs or carotid or vertebral artery bruits, and her lying and standing blood pressures were both 160/80.

Management

An X-ray of her cervical spine revealed that there was osteophyte formation which was particularly marked between the sixth and seventh vertebral bodies. Both an electroencephalogram and a tomogram of her head showed no abnormalities. A number of supraventricular extrasystoles were seen on a 24 hour recording of an electrocardiogram; none of these were associated with symptoms (Chapter 10, "Cardiac arrhythmias"), and the tracing was considered to be normal for a woman of her age.

Although the changes noted in the cervical vertebrae are common in old age, it was considered reasonable to assume, by a process of exclusion, that her "blackouts" were due to vertebrobasilar insufficiency, and she was put onto aspirin in a dose of 300 mg daily and fitted with a tight-fitting cervical collar. There has been no recurrence of her symptoms.

Review of her medical records revealed that X-ray of her lumbar spine had shown extensive osteoarthritis. She had been advised already to purchase a firm mattress. The physiotherapist organised a programme of exercises designed to strengthen her back muscles (Chapter 7, "Vertebral column").

When her thyroid function was checked, it emerged that her

plasma free thyroxine level was high at 30 pmol/l and her plasma thyroid-stimulating hormone level low at 0.1 μg/l (Chapter 13, "Hypothyroidism—Treatment"). This suggested that she was on too large a dose of thyroxine, and this was reduced to 50 μg daily.

Over the first few visits at the day hospital, more detailed questioning established that she felt tired most of the time, that she had difficulty in concentrating, and that she felt extremely lonely. Her appetite was poor, and she often experienced a churning feeling in her stomach. She sometimes hoped that she would not wake up in the morning, and admitted to having occasionally harboured thoughts about suicide. The diagnosis of depression was confirmed by the visiting psychiatrist, and she was put on to progressively increasing doses of lofepramine until this reached 70 mg in the morning and 140 mg each evening. Regular review showed that this did not produce drowsiness, confusion, ataxia or postural hypotension. Her mood improved over the subsequent 2 months when she was discharged from the day hospital.

CASE 7: FEMALE, AGED 72 YEARS

History

The patient had started smoking cigarettes while still at school. Some 30 years later she had a "smoker's cough" which over the years progressed to classical winter bronchitis. About 15 years previously she had had an uncomplicated myocardial infarction related to hypertension and coronary artery disease. Because of increasing shortness of breath her exercise tolerance had progressively decreased. Partly as a result of this her weight had increased quite rapidly. Chronic heart failure with atrial fibrillation had been diagnosed 5 years previously but was easily controlled with digoxin and diuretics. Two weeks before admission she had visited her GP because of pain in the knees which required anti-inflammatory analgesics and she had been advised to lose weight. Following this visit her breathing worsened rapidly, she developed an increased cough productive of green sputum and became severely confused. She was admitted as an emergency.

The patient was overweight, apathetic and depressed. She was nauseated, anorectic and variably confused. Mental test score on admission was 5/10 (Chapter 9). There was pitting oedema of the legs and sacrum, jugular veins were distended and pulsatile. The

Case 6.

Problems	Effects	Actions
Vertebrobasilar insufficiency	(i) Dizziness (ii) "Blackouts" (iii) Stroke	(a) Cervical collar (PT) (b) Aspirin (D) (c) Personal alarm (SW)
Osteoarthritis of lumbar spine	(i) Back pain (ii) Sciatica (iii) Poor mobility	(a) Back exercises (PT) (b) Firm mattress (D) (c) Walking exercises (PT)
Hypothyroidism	(i) Hypothermia (ii) Mental and physical slowness	(a) Ensure drug compliance (D, CN, PH) (b) Review dosage (D, GP)
Depression	(i) Self-neglect (ii) Poor nutrition (iii) Isolation (iv) Suicide	(a) Antidepressant (PG) (b) Advice/support (CPN) (c) Day hospital/centre (PG, OT, SW)

Key. CN = community nurse; CPN = community psychiatric nurse; D = doctor; GP = general practitioner; N = nurse; OT = occupational therapist; PG = psychogeriatrician; PH = pharmacist; PT = physiotherapist; SW = social worker.

heart was enlarged with normal heart sounds. The pulse was 70 beats per minute and irregular. The blood pressure was 160/90 mmHg. There were obvious signs of basal consolidation of the left lung and basal crepitations heard at the right base. Apart from mild deformity and crepitus in both knees the rest of her physical examination was normal.

Management

The sudden worsening of her previously controlled chronic cardiac failure was attributed to the effects of the recently prescribed non-steroidal anti-inflammatory drug (NSAID) for her osteoarthritis. The majority of NSAIDs, via their prostaglandin synthetase inhibitory activity, variably cause salt and water retention especially in elderly patients. Thus, they can exacerbate both chronic cardiac failure and hypertension. The cardiac failure was then made worse by the digoxin induced bradycardia. The absence of a tachycardia in a patient with deteriorating cardiac failure and a chest infection alerted the geriatrician who arranged for an emergency electrocardiogram (ECG). This showed atrial fibrillation, slow ventricular rate of 68/minute and ST changes typical of digoxin toxicity. The plasma digoxin level was later reported to have been 3.8 mmol/l, almost twice the upper limit of the therapeutic range. The combination of old age and chronic cardiac failure reduces glomerular filtration rate and decreases digoxin excretion (Chapter 13, "Renal function"). The addition of dehydration producing a pre-renal element was the final step which precipitated digoxin intoxication (Chapter 10, "Cardiac failure"). The digoxin was stopped and intravenous rehydration commenced. More urgent measures were not undertaken as her arrhythmia was not thought to be life threatening and dehydration was prominent. Antibiotics were given intravenously. Because of rapid improvement in her blood urea (32–15 mmol/l within 24 hours) it was concluded that dehydration was indeed pre-renal secondary to water loss from the breathlessness, pulmonary oedema and respiratory infection combined with a low fluid intake due to her relative immobility (Chapter 13, "Fluid balance"). During respiration dry air is taken in and saturated air is expired. In states of increased ventilation the net loss of water can be considerable. Similarly an immobilised patient may inhabit a water desert and have a markedly reduced fluid intake. Water has to be *prescribed* and monitored by nursing and medical staff.

Inability to maintain fluid intake at home during an acute illness is an important indication for hospital admission.

Her confusion rapidly resolved and was thought to be secondary to the digoxin and the toxic effects of her chest infection. Depression and confusion are common in elderly people with digoxin intoxication whereas the gastrointestinal features (anorexia/nausea) are less common. Blood gases did not show gross hypoxia or hypercapnia. The initial urinary incontinence rapidly resolved after treatment of the quite severe constipation (Chapter 14).

CASE 8: FEMALE, AGED 89 YEARS

History

A general practitioner sent a letter to a consultant geriatrician reporting that the patient had suffered from recurrent episodes of left mandibular pain over the last 4 months. These had occurred, on average, three times a week and had lasted about 30 minutes and 2 hours. There were no obvious precipitating factors.

An additional problem was that over the last 2 years she had suffered from urinary frequency, so that she had had to visit the lavatory every 45 minutes during the day, and had had to get up three times during the night. Over the last 3 weeks she had suffered from occasional episodes of urinary incontinence. The problem had been exacerbated by the fact that there had been a deterioration in her mobility. During the day, she was rather unsteady, but at night, required assistance to get up out of bed, and to get around the house.

She had moved in to live with her daughter and son-in-law after the death of her husband from myocardial infarction 3 years ago. The arrangement had worked well initially, but her son-in-law had become increasingly exasperated recently by the disruption of their social life, and the stress which caring for her mother had imposed upon his wife.

There was a previous history of depression requiring admission to a psychiatric hospital in 1967, and of treatment of congestive cardiac failure by her general practitioner since 1988.

Her current medication was bendrofluazide 5 mg daily, co-proxamol two tablets as required for pain, and temazepam 10 mg each evening for insomnia. She was also receiving quinine in a

Case 7.

Problems	Effects	Actions
Bronchitis Pneumonia	(i) Shortness of breath on exertion (ii) Dehydration (iii) Digoxin retention	(a) Test bronchodilators (D, PT) (b) Stop smoking (D, N) (c) Antibiotics (D) (d) Prescribe fluids, oral and intravenous (D, N)
Ischaemic heart disease	(i) Myocardial infarction (ii) Atrial fibrillation	(a) Digoxin and diuretics (D)
Hypertension	(i) Chronic cardiac failure	(a) Diuretics (D)
Osteoarthritis (OA) of knees	(i) Immobility (ii) Fluid retention	(a) Pain relief (D) (b) Physiotherapy (PT) (c) Weight reduction (DT)
NSAIDs	(i) Worsening chronic cardiac failure	(a) Withdraw (D) (b) Paracetamol (D)
Obesity	(i) Immobility (ii) Osteoarthritic knees	(a) Weight reduction (DT) (b) Re-mobilise (PT) (c) Paracetamol (D)
Digoxin intoxication	(i) Anorexia (ii) Constipation (iii) Depression (iv) Confusion	(a) Remove digoxin (D) (b) Rehydrate (N)

Key: DT = dietitian; D = doctor; N = nurse; PT = physiotherapist.

dose of 300 mg each evening for treatment of nocturnal cramps in her legs.

Examination

She exhibited little facial expression, and walked slowly with a shuffling gait. There was some increase in tone in all four limbs, but more marked on the left side. Although she did not have a tremor under baseline conditions, this could be induced by asking her to perform mental arithmetic.

Her pulse was regular and had a rate of 86 beats per minute, and her blood pressure was 140/85 mmHg. She had no jugular venous congestion, but had bilateral oedema of her feet and legs. The skin over her ankles was discoloured, shiny and atrophic, but there was no actual ulceration.

Management

She was referred to the day hospital for more detailed evaluation of her condition.

A dentist at the day hospital examined her mouth and gums to ensure that her facial pain was not due to a lesion such as root infection, but detected no abnormality. Although the symptoms were rather atypical for trigeminal neuralgia, she was started on carbamazepine in a dose of 50 mg daily. Despite this, she continued to suffer from bouts of facial pain, and sometimes this lasted all day. The possibility of psychogenic pain was considered, and she was given imipramine in a dose of 25 mg three times daily. This reduced the frequency and severity of the episodes.

The aetiology of lower limb oedema was reviewed (Table 10.4: Causes of lower leg oedema). An ultrasound probe produced evidence of deep venous thrombosis in both legs. In view of this bendrofluazide was discontinued and the physiotherapists treated the swelling with "Flotron" boots. Also she was measured for graded pressure elasticated stockings, but before these were fitted, an ultrasound probe was used to ensure that the arterial pressure in her calves was not reduced.

Since there were signs of early Parkinson's disease, and since this was affecting her mobility, it was decided to treat her (Chapter 8, "Parkinson's disease"). There is some evidence that dopamine agonists exert a protective effect on the neurones in the substantia nigra, and she was started, therefore, on amantadine in a dose of 100 mg daily, increasing after 2 weeks to 200 mg daily. Parallel with this she was given a course of physiotherapy which concentrated on increasing the length and height of her stride, and overcoming hesitancy associated with initiating walking or passing through a doorway.

It seemed likely that her cramps were related to Parkinson's disease, and quinine was discontinued. The cramps subsided once the dose of amantadine was stabilised.

The patient was reviewed by a nurse continence adviser, (Chapter 14 "Treatment") who identified severe atrophic vaginitis. Dual channel cystometrography showed that she had no residual urine, that her resting bladder pressure was 7 cm of water, that there were no spontaneous contractions and that the maximum bladder capacity was 650 ml. Dienoestrol cream, 0.01%, was prescribed, and arrangements made for a community nurse to apply this daily for 2 weeks, reducing this to three times a week for a further 3 months. This, combined with her improved mobility, stopping bendrofluazide and coincidental treatment with imipramine eliminated her incontinence.

Despite the improvement in her physical health, it was clear that the atmosphere at home remained strained. After considerable discussion, she and her daughter and son-in-law decided that the best option would be for her to move into private warden supported sheltered housing which had recently been erected in the neighbourhood. The move was extremely successful. Indeed within 6 weeks of the move her facial pain had disappeared, and it was possible to discontinue the imipramine.

CASE 9: MALE, AGED 72 YEARS

History

This retired carpenter had been referred to the geriatric medical outpatient clinic following 2 weeks of haemoptysis. The patient denied any other symptoms though direct questioning revealed that he had a productive morning cough of many years' duration, the result of 60 years' cigarette smoking. The patient was otherwise very fit and thought that his general practitioner was being unnecessarily cautious in arranging hospital investigation. As far

Case 8.

Problems	Effects	Actions
Facial pain	(i) Poor life quality (ii) Depression	(a) Diagnose and treat cause (D, DE)
Chronic venous insufficiency	(i) Oedema, eczema, leg ulcers (ii) Poor mobility	(a) Graded pressure stockings (PT) (b) "Flotron" boots (PT)
Parkinson's disease	(i) Poor mobility (ii) Self-care problems (iii) Problems with housework (iv) Falls (v) Mental impairment (vi) Depression (vii) Hypothermia (viii) Poor nutrition (ix) Dysarthria	(a) Drug treatment (D) (b) Walking exercises (PT) (c) Dressing practice (OT) (d) Adaptations to clothing and household (OT, SW) (e) Home help (SW) (f) Personal alarm (SW) (g) Central heating (HD) (h) Self help, advice (PDS) (i) Speech therapy (ST)
Urinary incontinence	(i) Embarrassment (ii) Carer stress (iii) Skin damage (iv) Institutionalisation	(a) Investigate and advise (CA) (b) Treat cause (D) (c) Toilet training (N) (d) Local surgery (G, U) (e) Marsupial pants, urinals etc. (N) (f) Laundry service (SW) (g) Special clothing (OT)
Tension between patient and relatives/carer	(i) Marital breakdown (ii) Elder abuse	(a) Increase support as above (b) Sheltered housing (HD) (c) Residential/nursing home

Key: CA = continence adviser; D = doctor; DE = dentist; G = gynaecologist; HD = housing department; PT = physiotherapist; OT = occupational therapist; PDS = Parkinson's Disease Society; ST = speech therapist; U = urologist; SW = social worker.

as the patient was concerned the only problem he had was his wife who suffered from a poor memory. As a result of this he had gradually assumed more and more responsibility for running the household, shopping and cooking. Apart from minimal signs of bronchitis (slightly over-distended chest and some pulmonary rhonchi) physical examination was normal. The chest X-ray showed a mediastinal round mass approximately 8 cm in diameter. Sputum cytology was negative and other routine investigations were entirely normal.

Management

He was admitted to the programmed investigation unit (Chapter 3, "Where should investigations be done?"). Two early morning sputum samples were sent to the microbiology laboratory for microscopy and culture to exclude tuberculosis. Pulmonary function studies were surprisingly good in spite of his underlying smoking-induced chronic bronchitis. It is important to confirm respiratory function before submitting patients to bronchoscopy (Chapter 3, "Other investigations"). Bronchoscopy showed an ulcerated tumour partially blocking the right main bronchus. The carina was not widened. Biopsy subsequently revealed the typical cytological features of small cell cancer. The situation was discussed with the patient (Chapter 15, "What to tell the patient"). He was adamant that his wife nor indeed anyone else should be told the diagnosis. His "performance status" was good (normal serum lactate dehydrogenase, albumin, alkaline phosphatase and sodium). He was offered the opportunity of active treatment (chemotherapy) at this stage. The various options with their pros and cons were presented to him and discussed on a number of occasions by different members of staff. It proved easy to be "free and frank", which is very necessary if the patient is going to make an informed decision. His main concern was for his wife. After a few days' reflection he decided against chemotherapy. He was introduced to the Macmillan (cancer) nurse specialist who arranged to visit him at home (Chapter 4, "Community services"). Further investigations (bone scan, abdominal and cerebral CT) were not performed as the decision not to undertake active treatment had been agreed. A full report, including what the patient had been told, was sent to the general practitioner. The linchpin of successful "shared care" between hospital and the general practice team depends on accurate and rapid communication. Three weeks later the Macmillan nurse reported back to the geriatric unit that the patient had quite suddenly deteriorated—he had lost his appetite and had become aggressive and uncooperative. Assessment in the outpatient department showed that his physical condition apart from a 1 kg weight loss was unchanged but he had other signs of depression. He was not obviously suicidal and could therefore be treated at home which was advantageous to his wife. It was decided that the Macmillan nurse visiting would be increased and he was prescribed fluoxetine, a rapidly acting 5-hydroxytryptamine (5-HT) uptake inhibitor (Chapter 9, "Depression"). Over the course of the next few weeks he improved considerably. The association of depression with physical disability is common in elderly patients and is always worth treating. He remained well for a further 3 months until he quite suddenly became confused and drowsy.

He was rapidly admitted to the geriatric acute assessment ward where a right basal pneumonia was confirmed. There were no neurological signs apart from drowsiness and quite severe confusion. Before starting treatment an urgent CT scan was carried out to exclude cerebral metastases. If these had been found the decision to continue active treatment would have been different. He was rehydrated parenterally and prescribed antibiotics. His confusion resolved within 36 hours and by day 3 he was ready to go home. Unfortunately while remobilising he experienced a sudden onset of severe and persistent haemoptysis which frightened both the patient and his wife. He was reviewed by the local radiotherapist who arranged for a single 8 Gy fraction treatment instead of a conventional concentrated 10 day course of 30 Gy. This allowed treatment to be completed at a single visit to the oncology centre.

He returned home but obviously was not as capable of managing the house and his wife unaided as he was before. The social worker arranged for a home help on a twice weekly basis and an Age Concern "shopper" helped regularly (Chapter 4, "Community services"). The Macmillan nurse developed a close relationship and it was she who raised the problem of terminal care with the patient and discussed various options. The wife was not party to these discussions which complicated matters. The patient was not at ease with the idea of hospice care even after he had visited the local one in company with "his" Macmillan nurse. It was decided that if the general practitioner and the Macmillan nurse could not manage at home then he would prefer to be admitted to the local geriatric unit.

This arrangement was agreed by all and an assurance given that admission would be guaranteed by the geriatric unit "on demand" by the general practitioner, the nurse or the patient himself. In the event he went rapidly downhill and was admitted with pneumonia. No antibiotics or infusion were given on this occasion. Sedatives in gradually increasing doses were given for breathlessness and he died peacefully 72 hours after admission. During one of his infrequent lucid periods he thanked "his" Macmillan nurse and said goodbye to her.

CASE 10: MALE, AGED 84 YEARS

History

The patient was referred to an outpatient clinic. He had been on treatment for Parkinson's disease for 6 years. Over the last 6 weeks he had become increasingly tired, and found that even the effort of dressing made him breathless. An additional problem was that over the last 4 weeks he had noticed that solid foods had tended to stick in his gullet.

He had suffered from pain in his knees for 4 years, and was currently on 400 mg of ibuprofen three times daily for this. In 1984 he had had a transurethral prostatectomy. This had left him with urinary incontinence, and over the last 3 years he had been fitted with a urinary catheter.

He lived in a three bedroom bungalow with his wife who was 76 years old and was in good health.

Examination

He was of spare build and his conjunctivae were extremely pale. He had some jugular venous congestion, a few coarse crepitations at both lung bases, and a trace of oedema at both ankles. His pulse was regular with a rate of 102 beats per minute, and there was a pansystolic murmur at his apex conducted into his axilla. There was osteophyte formation around both knee joints, and there was crepitus and pain on passive movement. He walked with a shuffling gait but there was no rigidity or tremor. More prolonged observation revealed that there were times when he developed a mild orofacial dyskinesia.

Case 9.

Problems	Effects	Actions
Chronic bronchitis	Cough	(a) Stop smoking (GP) (b) Treat infections (GP)
Haemoptysis	Fear	(a) Investigate cause (D) (rarely due to bronchitis) (b) Radiotherapy (R)
Carcinoma of lung	(i) Haemoptysis and other symptoms (ii) Weight loss	(a) Diagnose (D) (b) Type/stage/complications (D) (c) Specific treatment (D) (d) Treat symptoms (D) (e) Support (GP, D, MN)
Complications	(i) Depression	(a) Treat (D) (b) Counsel and support (MN, GP, D)
"Confused" wife	(i) Dependency	(a) Diagnosis (GP) (b) Support (SW) (c) Refer to PG (GP)

Key: D = doctor; GP = general practitioner; MN = Macmillan nurse; R = radiotherapist; PG = psychogeriatrician; SW = social worker.

Management

A chest X-ray confirmed that there was cardiomegaly, that he had prominent pulmonary vascular markings and that there was diversion of blood to the upper lobes. He was treated with frusemide in a dose of 40 mg daily, and this produced rapid resolution of the signs of failure.

Examination of a blood sample showed that he had a haemoglobin of 7.7 g/dl, and that the red cells were hypochromic and microcytic. Once his cardiac failure had been controlled he was transfused with four units of packed cells, 20 mg frusemide being given intravenously with each unit, and a careful watch was kept for signs of cardiac failure. His haemoglobin increased to 10.4 g/dl and his symptoms of tiredness and lethargy disappeared following the transfusion (Chapter 12, "Anaemia").

A barium swallow identified an area of narrowing and irregularity at the lower end of the oesophagus. This was followed by endoscopy at which an ulcerated tumour was visualised. A biopsy established that this was a poorly differentiated adenocarcinoma.

The diagnosis was discussed with the patient and his wife. They accepted the advice that the most appropriate option was palliative surgery. He was transferred to an adjacent cardiothoracic surgical unit where a thoracotomy was performed, and a Celestin tube passed through the area of stenosis and fixed in position. The patient made a good recovery from the operation (Chapter 12, "Dysphagia").

His Parkinson's disease (Chapter 8) was treated with the L-dopa/benserazide combination Madopar in a dose of 125 mg four times daily. In view of the history of gastrointestinal blood loss it was decided not to treat his osteoarthritis with NSAIDs, and he was prescribed paracetamol in a dose of 1 g four times daily. After a short programme of walking exercises he regained his mobility and was discharged home.

He remained in reasonable health for 4 months, but then he began to lose weight and developed severe abdominal discomfort. He was readmitted and examination revealed that his liver was enlarged. It was firm, but no discrete nodules were palpated. Ultrasonography established that the liver contained multiple tumours.

Because he was in considerable distress, he was put on to a 4 hourly mixture containing 2.5 mg of morphine. This was later increased to 5 mg 4 hourly, and finally changed to pump infusion

Case 10.

Problems	Effects	Actions
Congestive cardiac failure	(i) Breathlessness (ii) Peripheral oedema	(a) Diuretics, ACE inhibitors (D)
Anaemia	(i) Lethargy, cardiac failure etc.	(a) Haematinic (D) (b) Blood transfusion (D)
Carcinoma of oesophagus	(i) Dysphagia (ii) Anaemia (iii) Poor nutrition (iv) Metastatic disease (v) Anxiety	(a) Radical or palliative surgery (S) (b) Nutrient supplements (N) (c) Good communication with patient and relatives (D, N, SW) (d) Counselling (GP, D, N, SW)
Osteoarthritis	(i) Immobility (ii) Pain	(a) Walking exercises (PT) (b) Analgesics (D) (c) Walking aids (PT) (d) Joint replacement (OS)
Parkinson's disease (see Case 8)	(i) Immobility	(a) L-dopa therapy (D)
Terminal pain	(i) Poor quality death (ii) Anxiety	(a) Effective analgesia (D) (b) Communication and counselling—?Tranquilliser (D, GP, N, SW, C)
Death	(i) Spouse's bereavement	(a) Good communication with GP and bereaved (D) (b) Further support by GP (CN, HV)

Key: C = clergyman; CN = community nurse; D = doctor; HV = health visitor; GP = general practitioner; PT = physiotherapist; OS = orthopaedic surgeon; S = surgeon; SW = social worker.

of 30 mg of diamorphine every 24 hours. This kept his discomfort under control and he died 6 days later (Chapter 15, "Relief of symptoms").

CHAPTER 1 Demography and population statistics

The increase in the proportion of old people in society is a relatively recent phenomenon. The process has been simmering since prehistory, but the full impact has only become apparent in the present century (Figure 1.1). The highest proportions of old people are to be found in the so-called developed nations, mostly situated in the northern hemisphere. But it is important to realise that the growth of the elderly population will be the fastest of any age group (including children) in Africa, Latin America and South East Asia during the next two decades. Thus, throughout the world, the number of people over the age of 60 years will increase by over 100% during this period.

This change in population structure is not due, in the main, to the old living longer, but because fewer younger and middle-aged people are dying. Figure 1.2 differentiates, in a statistical way, between deaths due to accidents and disease, and senescent deaths due to inevitable ageing. Better public health (including health education and health promotion), social improvements, better nutrition and, recently, medical advances have reduced the premature mortality rate. Thus, life expectancy for a boy in the United Kingdom in 1986 was 71.9 years, and for a girl 77.7 years.

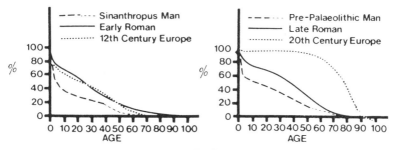

Figure 1.1 Survival curves through the ages

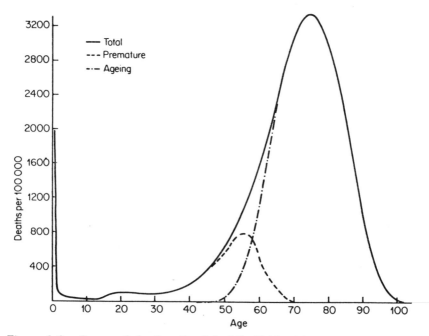

Figure 1.2 Curve of deaths, English Life Table 13, 1970–1972; men (from OPCS, 1980, © Crown copyright, by permission of the Controller of HMSO)

A more recently recognised phenomenon has been a rise in the life expectancy of older people. Table 1.1 suggests that the increase in expectation of life is occurring in each quinquennial age group, and that it has been slightly greater for men aged 65 and 70 than for women. This is something which is happening gradually and is occurring world-wide, for during the period 1955 too 1986 life

Table 1.1 Change in life expectation for age groups of men and women in the United Kingdom between 1978–1980 and 1987–1989 (*Annual Abstract of Statistics*, 1992)

Age in years	Males (life expectancy in years)		Females (life expectancy in years)	
	1978–1980	1987–1980	1978–1980	1987–1989
65	12.6	13.8	16.6	17.6
70	9.7	10.8	13.0	14.0
75	7.4	8.3	9.8	10.8
80	5.6	6.3	7.2	8.0
85+	4.1	4.7	5.1	5.8

expectation for a 65-year-old man increased from 11.8 years to 13.4 years, and from 14.8 years to 17.3 years for a 65-year-old woman. In Japan the increase over the same period has been even greater, the figures being from 11.8 years to 15.9 years in men and from 14.1 years to 19.3 years in women:

The reason for this pattern is not clear, but, as Table 1.2 shows, death rates for decennial groups of elderly have fallen in the 1980s and the gap between men and women is narrowing. Factors such as intensive health education at the workplace, better nutrition, and less poverty may play a part. It is likely though, that the phenomenon of increasing life expectation at birth as a result of "medical" and "social" advances is subject to the law of diminishing returns. Thus, with the exception of cardiovascular diseases, abolition of disease (including cancer) would have but a minimal effect on the average expection of life. The survival curve (Figure 1.1) is now almost rectilinear.

By the turn of the century, the *world* population over the age of 60 years will have reached 580 million, a 60% increase over 25 years. Two-thirds of these people will live in the *less-developed* regions. Thus, nearly one in ten individuals will be over the age of 60 years. The socio-economic consequences of this are enormous as are those which relate to health service planning and provision. Only these latter aspects will be examined. Table 1.3 shows the estimated population projections for the 40 year period 1991 to 2031. As can be seen there will be little increase in the total number over 65 years until the year 2011. However, the numbers of those over 80 and 85 years will continue to grow and it is these age groups that will pose the greatest challenge to both medical and social services. It should be noted also that the female : male ratio changes from its present level of 1 : 3 to 1 : 2.

Table 1.2   Death rates per 1000 population 1981 and 1990 (UK) (*Annual Abstract of Statistics,* 1992)

	Age	65–74	75–84	Over 85
1981	M	47.5	110.6	239.5
	F	25.5	70.4	190.6
1990	M	39.5	94.3	187.8
	F	22.4	58.9	156.7

Table 1.3   Population projections for the United Kingdom 1991–2031 by age groups (source: *Annual Abstract of Statistics*, 1992)

| | Age | Thousands | | | | |
		65–74	75–79	80–84	Over 85 years	Total
1991	M	2258	720	422	224	3624
	F	2770	1130	839	668	5407
	T	5028	1850	1261	892	9031
2001	M	2237	799	476	317	3829
	F	2574	1127	843	853	5397
	T	4811	1926	1319	1170	9226
2011	M	2472	791	532	410	4205
	F	2763	1030	840	827	5460
	T	5235	1821	1372	1237	9665
2021	M	2876	948	565	452	4841
	F	3245	1204	841	899	6189
	T	6121	2152	1406	1351	11030
2031	M	3281	1006	751	536	5574
	F	3646	1281	1113	1002	7042
	T	6927	2287	1864	1538	12616

HEALTH OF THE ELDERLY

Most elderly people are healthy in both body and mind, and even those who survive into extreme old age lead an independent, unsupported way of life for most of this period. They should be encouraged and, if need be, assisted to continue in this way, though it may be necessary to orchestrate health and social services to enable them to do so (Chapter 4). The Darwinian theory of the "Survival of the Fittest" is to a certain extent true of the oldest old, those who are in their nineties or who become centenarians. Many are in better health than individuals ten years their junior. They have been termed the "biological elite" (Case 5), though genetic inheritance, lifestyle, and environmental factors particularly in early life, or even *in utero*, may have played a part.

In terms of the measurement of the state of a person's health chronological age is relatively unimportant. Within each elderly age group there are people who have normal physiological parameters, while others have disability-associated pathological changes within organs and abnormal physiological responses. This may or may not affect their capacity to lead independent lives of a quality which they find satisfactory. Individuals in good health have been termed the "young old" whereas those who are dependent on help, of varying degrees, for their continuing survival have been called the "old old". Alternatively the terms "Third Age" and "Fourth Age" have been used.

Though chronological age has relatively little effect on the degree of "oldness" or "age", it would be foolish to suggest that time has no effect on the ageing process. Indeed the basic concept of ageing is loss with time of the organism's adaptability to internal and external stress. Various mechanisms and theories have been proposed to account for human ageing. Because of their complexity, it has been suggested that these theories probably obscure the problem! Any theory must satisfy four criteria—the process must be intrinsic, deleterious, progressive and universal to the species. The most persuasive theory proposed is the disposable stroma mechanism, which suggests that many of the features of ageing result from the inability of body cells to repair random environmental damage. The rate at which ageing occurs will depend on the variability of these external events as well as genetically determined repair factors. This theory need not be exclusive of others.

While ageing alters organ function and physiology and leads to some decline in physical, mental, and social capacity, the effect often only becomes apparent when there is a medical or social crisis. Some old people take a negative view of life leading to the

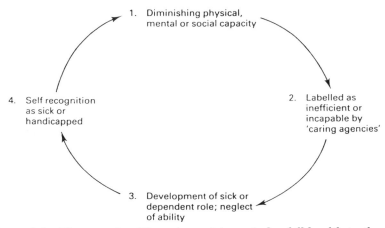

Figure 1.3   The negative life cycle: a vicious circle of ill health in the elderly

adoption of a negative life cycle (Figure 1.3), and may go on to develop a sick and dependent role. This descending spiral of diminishing ability may be reinforced by well-meaning relatives or even some caring professionals (Chapter 4). A positive life cycle (Figure 1.4) requires excitement, risk and even danger. It also requires the recognition of this fact by health professionals and society generally.

Unfortunately, ill health, disease and disability increase with increasing age. This is not entirely surprising if one remembers that most diseases are the result of some interaction between the individual and the environment, and the longer someone is exposed to risk, the higher the probability of a pernicious interaction. Recent longitudinal population studies confirm an exponential increase in morbidity with increasing age, starting in late middle life.

In general terms, just over 15% of the United Kingdom (UK) population is aged 65 years or more and this figure will remain constant until 2011 (Table 1.3). Thus, in a standard population of 10 000 people of all ages, 1566 will be over the age of 65 years, and of these only 72 (4.6%) will be in an institution (hospital, nursing home or old people's home) at any one time. The vast majority (95.4%) live in their own homes or in "homely" settings

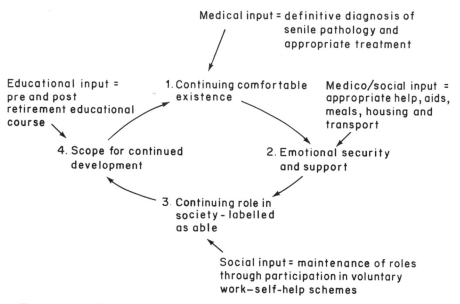

Figure 1.4   The positive life cycle

in the community. Nevertheless within this population of people over 65 years of age there is a marked age-related institutionalisation rate. Thus, half of all individuals over 95 years of age are in institutions at any one time. The proportion of old people in institutions varies from country to country and also within countries. Attitudes of authorities vary, such as in Scotland where, twenty years ago, the "norm" for geriatric hospital bed numbers was 15/1000 elderly as opposed to 10/1000 elderly in England and Wales. That these figures bore no real relation to actual need, or provision, in some places has perhaps hindered the development of the overall care of the elderly. Until the publication of the White Paper "Caring for People" (1989) and the Audit Commission Reports (1985 and 1986) that preceded it, a fifth of the institutionalised elderly were in hospital. The remainder were divided between local authority (LA) residential homes (40%) and nursing (10%) or residential homes run by private (20%) or voluntary agencies (10%).

Since the mid-1980s a considerable change has taken place. Local authorities have recognised that residential care is an expensive way of providing support and care for a small number of people, and that better use could be made of the money available if homes were closed. At the same time the government encouraged the growth of the private sector by widening the Board and Lodging allowances to include Income Support for elderly people in residential homes or nursing homes, and who were unable to meet the cost. This has meant Income Support expenditure, which totalled £10 million in 1979/80, had risen to £774 million in 1987/88 and now exceeds £1 billion, being claimed by approximately 1.4 million pensioners in 1990. In the same period the cost of Attendance Allowance and Invalid Care Allowance rose from £205 million to £1081 million—a real terms increase of 200%.

Similarly, since in 1993 the long-term care of the elderly becomes the responsibility of LA social service departments, health authorities have been studying their needs in terms of hospital beds. Every health service has difficulty matching resources to need, not primarily because of financial straits, although these are obviously important, but rather because of lack of hard data. In the past, disability (not need) has often been the reason for placement in an institution. Yet 58% of the most severely disabled and dependent people, including some who are bedfast, remain in the community and not in hospital (Table 1.4). These figures are generalised aggregates and each area needs to collect its own information if it is to plan and to provide a service for old people. Equally, planning requires coordination of both hospital and community care—neither can plan or work in isolation. Recent government legislation (NHS and Community Care Act 1990) placed the responsibility for "Continuing Care" on the LA social services departments. It directed that each LA region should draw up a Community Care Plan by April 1992 and that the accent to be placed on "Community Care" should aim at maximising the proportion of disadvantaged people living outside institutions. This would involve a reassessment of *needs* and the development of objectives and priorities. Included amongst the "disadvantaged" are those who suffer infirmity or mental illness in old age. In order to achieve this LAs have had to consult widely, including not only health authorities (HA) but also housing authorities, voluntary agencies and the private sector in order to make arrangements for coordinating care. This has meant creating service agreements, improving information systems and arrangements to secure quality. At the time of writing few plans are finalised and comment is difficult. But, the objective is to set up a user-centred, cost effective seamless system of community-based health and care services.

HEALTH SERVICES FOR THE ELDERLY

The elderly use approximately half of all the hospital facilities in the United Kingdom, and as the population ages and increases so will this usage. They consume about a quarter of all prescribed drugs and use more than a third of the resources of primary care teams (general practitioners). The demographic changes already outlined are the main reason for escalating health costs.

It has long been recognised that while the cost of treatment in

Table 1.4   Disability and residence: 1566 people over 65 years

Function level	Home No. (%)	Institution No. (%)	Total No. (%)
Bedfast	28 (58)	20 (42)	48 (3)
Confined to "house"	162 (91)	17 (9)	179 (11)
Mobile with "aid"	121 (90)	14 (10)	135 (9)
Independent	1181 (98)	23 (2)	1204 (77)
Total	1494 (95)	72 (5)	1566 (100)

a geriatric bed per day is somewhat less than that in general ward, the cost per inpatient stay may be four times as expensive. A clear need to reduce length of hospital stay exists. To achieve this, disability must be prevented and independence increased. For this reason, while the use of high technology medicine may be individually expensive, if used appropriately, even in the very old, it is cost effective in terms of early diagnosis, effective treatment, and prevention or amelioration of dependency and disability. Accurate diagnosis of pathological change and assessment of physiological state enables an effective treatment plan to be instituted. Treatment options and plans need to be fully discussed with patients and sometimes with their relatives.

COMMUNITY CARE

The successful management of an ill, elderly person depends upon a rapid response from the primary health care team—delay in meeting the medical needs can lead to accelerated physical, mental or social deterioration, and to the development of semi-permanent dependency. The difficulties of accurate clinical diagnosis and evaluation are outlined throughout this book. This, however, is not to deny the skilled role of other health professionals in the primary health care team. Thus, as can be seen from the case histories, the district nurse, health visitor, and social worker as well as the practice nurse and receptionist all have a very important part to play in the location, overall management and skilled support and treatment of ill old people. The primary health care team must be led by a skilled general practitioner for early diagnosis and management of ill health in the elderly cannot be delegated to non-physicians. It is common practice, now, for one doctor, in the larger group practices, to "specialise" in the "care of the elderly". Some of these doctors hold the Diploma of Geriatric Medicine of the Royal College of Physicians of London or the Royal College of Physicians and Surgeons of Glasgow.

One of the most difficult problems facing the primary health care team is "ascertainment". Old people tend to be stoical in their acceptance of disease and increasing disability. This attitude may also be reinforced, unfortunately, by well-meaning relatives who attribute symptoms and signs of disease to old age rather than to disease (Chapter 6). It is important that this "iceberg" of disease, most of which is remediable at an early stage, be uncovered by the primary health care team. In order to carry this out the team need a computerised age/sex register and the responsibility for obtaining this lies with the Family Health Services Authority (FHSA). Recent legislation requires the general practitioner to examine all elderly individuals over 75 years on a yearly basis. Using the register all such patients can be recorded as well as those who are "at risk", the latter being visited on a more frequent regular basis by the health visitor or district nurse. Primary health care teams are also encouraged to promote health, and many run well-person clinics at their surgeries, inviting their patients to attend on a voluntary basis. Such "screening" helps to disclose early ill health, though it is doubtful if screening is as valuable as "case finding". Nevertheless, the earlier symptomatic ill health can be treated the higher the probability of maintaining health and activity. Health education of the elderly to encourage early medical attention could be developed to a much greater extent.

Activity and a positive outlook to life must be encouraged. Many elderly have savings and use these for holidays which involve them in travel by air, sea and road. On reaching their destination they may experience environmental and physical hazards which have not been anticipated and which may trigger ill health. This means that they require advice before travelling abroad, and the general practitioner and his team often have the opportunity to do this when patients contact the surgery for information about immunisation when making plans.

The general practitioner often needs to call upon specialised resources—these may be the specialist in geriatric medicine, the psychogeriatrician or another health professional specialising in the care of the elderly. However, old people should not be disenfranchised from other specialist medical services such as cardiology, neurology, respirology, etc. In no way can the specialty of geriatric medicine provide overall medical care for all old people—nor would this be a beneficial development. The geriatrician has an important role in providing back-up skills to enable other specialists to discharge their elderly patients back into the community.

HOSPITAL SERVICES

Most departments of geriatric medicine in the United Kingdom are organised on progressive patient care lines. Basically each department should provide acute care wards (for assessment and treatment of acute illness), a rehabilitation service (either combined or separate from the acute wards) and a limited continuing care facility. To function properly the department of geriatric medicine must be located within the district general hospital (DGH) close by all diagnostic and treatment facilities. It also needs to provide a comprehensive outpatient service and, where appropriate, a domiciliary consultative service. Most departments also provide an outpatient rehabilitation service using a geriatric day hospital and some even supervise domiciliary teams of remedial therapists.

Acute Assessment

All elderly patients should have the benefit of a full medical work-up (Chapter 2 and 3). Certainly, no patient should be considered or accepted for long-term care, wherever finally placed, without the most careful and fullest investigation. The only difference between an acute geriatric medical ward and that of general or internal medicine is the greater emphasis on functional and performance aspects of disability within the geriatric area. In both types of ward the investigatory methods used to achieve a diagnosis, treatment and clinical management should be identical and based on the physical (physiological), mental and social state of the patient. The vast majority of the admissions to the acute geriatric ward should be from the community with the patients being returned there, after treatment, usually within the period of two weeks. Since it is impossible to separate acute illness from disability, acute units must be supported by the full rehabilitation team described in the next section.

Rehabilitation

A number of people admitted to acute wards (geriatric, surgical or medical) will, after treatment of their acute precipitating condition, require further physical rehabilitation. This is best carried out in a suitable environment orientated towards the slower progress of such individuals. Rehabilitation patients do not do well in the atmosphere of the acute ward, which may have to admit patients day and night. Though medical management of patients in rehabilitation wards needs to be continued, greater emphasis must be placed on remedial therapy. For this a fully trained team of integrated remedial therapists (physiotherapists, occupational therapists, speech therapists) is required. The ward nurses also are important members of this rehabilitation team and need to work closely with the therapists in a coordinated plan. In this environment, the old patient with, for example, a stroke (Chapter 8) can be retrained to maximise his potential ability and overcome or adapt to his disability. In many cases this rehabilitation programme makes the difference between long-term dependent care in an institution and living with residual disability and maximum function in the community. While the team of remedial therapists is based in the hospital and may initiate treatment in the rehabilitation ward, suitable subjects are frequently discharged early to their own homes and treatment continued on an outreach basis by the team. Recent developments now emphasise more community-based than hospital-based therapy. Many geriatric units have responded to the special needs of elderly patients sustaining injuries, such as a fractured proximal femur, by collaborating with orthopaedic surgeons to establish an orthogeriatric unit or service. The separate unit may be under the control of the geriatrician but have input from an orthopaedic surgeon, and have full back-up of the team of remedial therapists and social worker.

Continuing Care

There are a number of patients who do not respond to rehabilitation and for whom further care in some form of "caring home" is necessary. In the main this is due to the extreme disability produced by serious diseases, or, in comparatively rare cases, severe debility and frailty associated with extreme old age. Unfortunately, in a minority of cases this dependency may have been induced by inadequate care—either by physicians, other doctors, nurses and other carers (including relatives), or poor motivation from the patients, which in some instances may be the effect of depressive illness (Chapter 6). In these cases, slowness to act may have arisen at the outset of the disease, or from unawareness, until too late, of the subtle signs of disease (Chapter 2). Such disabled individuals need long-term nursing support, which is best accomplished outside the DGH, for in that setting such patients often get the label of failure attached to them with all its negative connotations. Unfortunately, however, long-term care in the NHS has been poorly developed, with some notable exceptions. (For further comment, see Chapter 4, "Long-term hospital care").

Psychogeriatric Care

Because of the high incidence and prevalence of psychiatric disease in older people, each geriatric unit needs to work in close association with a psychiatrist who has special responsibility for the elderly. Ideally, the psychogeriatric and geriatric units should be in close geographical relationship within the district general hospital to allow easy collaboration, cross-consultation, and, when necessary, joint case management. It is important for the psychogeriatric service to cover the whole field of mental illness in the elderly and not become just a dementia service. Affective disorders and neuroses are common, often coexisting with or being potentiated by physical illness and disability. Prompt and effective therapy can speed rehabilitation and develop independence, allowing earlier discharge home. The close liaison between geriatric and psychogeriatric services may be accomplished by joint sharing of some beds, although this is not uniformly essential. To achieve good collaboration, both services must have adequate resources; otherwise one service may become overprotective of its facilities and fail to cooperate effectively. Perhaps the ideal organisation is the creation of a joint department that combines both the medical and psychiatric aspects of the health care of the elderly. Such close integration is, however, difficult to achieve.

A psychogeriatric service needs day care places, outpatient sessions and staff to provide community back-up addition to beds in the hospital. Close links have to be forged with the primary health care team as well as social services and those providing residential care in the community. The community psychiatric nurse (CPN) has an important role to play in the support of patients and, equally importantly, their relatives and carers especially in those cases when the patient is severely disabled by dementia.

Organisational Models of Care

Whilst the progressive patient care model is the commonest scheme of geriatric care in the United Kingdom other models have and are being developed. Recent legislation will no doubt be a spur to further thinking on the most effective way of providing a comprehensive service to those elderly in need, for the geriatric service is likely to become the provider of a service, having a service agreement with a service commissioner (purchaser). In some areas the geriatric service will provide a comprehensive and exclusive medical service for all individuals over a certain age. At present, this usually is determined by the allocation of resources between general (internal) and geriatric medicine. In a few areas acute resources are shared equally between the two divisions, with the geriatrician (physician with an interest in geriatric medicine) playing a full part in a general medical service and, in addition, providing a geriatric rehabilitation and continuing-care service for the elderly. In many units in Scotland admission to a geriatric unit is dependent upon the needs as well as the age of the patient. Examples of patients with particular needs include those with multiple pathology, severe physical incapacity and an acute confusional state. A final model, common in Scandinavia, is for the geriatrician to be a specialist in long-term continuing care, with no commitment to acute clinical work, nor even to rehabilitation. Most geriatric services used to be described as hospital departments of geriatric medicine. Some practitioners, patients and relatives, however, felt that the word "geriatric" had pejorative connotations, so the title of the service was altered to "Department of Medicine for the Elderly", "Health Care of the Elderly Unit" or some similar variation. This should not alter the remit of the department!

Costs of Care

Mention has already been made of cost in relation to community care. All hospital care is expensive, and it has already been emphasised that geriatric hospital care is extremely expensive on a case cost basis. In 1990–1991 the annual cost to the Hospital and Community Health Service for elderly people aged 75 years and over averaged £1300 per head. The cost to the Family Health Service (FHS) was £270 per head and Social Services £500 per head. The geriatric service must be proactive and cost-effective if the health needs of the increasing numbers of the over 75 year age group are to be contained. Long stay residential care of all types for disabled and dependent elderly must be kept to a minimum. To achieve this, disability must be prevented or ameliorated at an early stage by expert medical and rehabilitative therapy. Additionally more disabled people and their carers should be supported and looked after in their own homes. This latter option is in line with current government policy, but it must be appreciated that the burden already borne by relatives and other non-professionals will be increased, as will the work of the primary health care teams. The current solution to this problem is for "integrated commissioning through care management". Some systems of care have already evolved which aim at keeping disabled and dependent elderly at home. For example, hospital teams are providing short-term care to the elderly at home, thereby supporting the primary health care team, organisation of care by the provision of day hospital attendance, short-term admission for a "holiday" or intermittently on a regular basis ("shared care") to give carers relief on a planned or semi-structured basis, as well as maintaining optimum function in the patient. In these ways long stay places can be kept to a minimum and resources used efficiently. Nevertheless the extra work placed on the hospital staff must be recognised.

FURTHER READING

Andrews, K. and Brocklehurst, J. (1987). *British Geriatric Medicine in the 1980's*. London: King Edward's Hospital Fund for London.

Audit Commission (1992). *Community Care: Managing the Cascade of Change*. London: HMSO.

Davies, B., Bebbington, A. and Charnley, H. *et al.* (1990). *Resources, Needs and Outcomes in Community-Based Care*. Aldershot: Avebury.

Denham, M.J. (1991). *Care of the Long-stay Elderly Patient, (2nd Edition)*. London: Chapman & Hall.

McIntosh, I.B. (1992). *Travel and Health in the Elderly: A Medical Handbook*. Lancaster: Quay.

Wells, N. and Freer, C. (Eds) (1988). *The Ageing Population. Burden or Challenge*. London: Macmillan.

CHAPTER 2 The elderly patient and his clinical problems

It often has been asked "What is so different about the geriatric patient? He is only you or I a little older." This is only true up to a point, for many differences do exist between the elderly patient and his younger counterparts. The objective of this chapter is to emphasise the differences as well as the similarities.

ADMISSION TO HOSPITAL

For many elderly patients, admission to a geriatric ward is their first experience of hospital, while others may not have been in hospital for many years. Consequently, their knowledge and image of hospital may be totally false, being coloured by what they have heard or previously experienced. This applies particularly to patients coming into the geriatric ward, since this often is considered to be little more than the last resting place prior to death. The evolution of modern hospitals and their geriatric units from old workhouses to their present day excellence within the life-time of old people may not be fully appreciated by the individual concerned.

For these reasons patients require reassurance and careful explanation of the function of the ward and what will happen to them. This assurance and explanation needs to be reinforced and repeated by all staff, not only doctors and nurses but also domestic staff whose importance in relation to patient care is often ignored or forgotten. The consultant under whose care the patient is admitted will often have begun this process if the patient has been seen before admission in the outpatient clinic or as a domiciliary visit. If this has not happened then the task should be initiated by members of the primary health care team, careful explanation being given to patients and their relatives when this is possible. If a patient is to be transferred from another hospital ward or hospital, then an explanation should be given not only by the geriatric staff when they see the patient in consultation, but also by the staff of the transferring ward. If possible, in these cases, the patient should be visited and seen by the nurse in charge of the receiving ward before transfer. The relatives must be told before the transfer occurs. The reason for the transfer should be made clear to the patient and relatives, and both disabused of the notion that geriatric care equates with long-term care.

The primary objective with elderly patients admitted to a geriatric ward must be to enable them to resume their place in society and the community as quickly as possible, so that the emphasis is on the rapid attainment of self-sufficiency. Since patients are encouraged to get up and dress as soon as possible, they should bring their clothes with them. Whenever possible, patients should be allowed to return to their homes at weekends; 5-days-a-week treatment and care experiments have already been performed with success.

THE ELDERLY PATIENT AS AN INDIVIDUAL

With the elderly, the doctor/nurse/patient relationship is different from most other groups, for a gap of at least one and sometimes two or three generations exists. Whereas the senior doctor is regarded as a father or companion figure by many of his patients, to the elderly he represents a "son" or a "grandson". While it is very good for the ego of the 50-year-old professor to be addressed as "boy", he and all others need to exhibit great tact and competence if they are to gain the respect and confidence of their elderly patient. Since hospital staff are strangers they have an advantage in this respect, but, initially, they will be treated with suspicion and must exercise caution and restraint in their management of the patient. There is no doubt that many elderly people are afraid of "being mucked about" or "experimented with" in hospital, but if the reasons for procedures are fully explained, together with the risks, there are few patients who are more cooperative and reasonable. Generally speaking, the elderly patient is one of the most rewarding of all patients to treat, for his expectation of gain is low and he responds gratefully to care, patience and skilled attention.

In order to understand their patients, all hospital staff must have some knowledge of the ageing process and the type of person that the patient has been. Here the hospital doctor may be at a disadvantage when compared to the family doctor who has probably known the patient over many years. It is vital that those based in hospital ensure that they collect any relevant information from the family doctor. For example, the following conversation took place one day:

Nurse (on telephone to resident doctor): "Dr Green, your patient Mrs Harris, who has just been admitted, is terribly confused. Will you please come and see her and write her up for a sedative?"

Dr Green: "How do you mean? Is she noisy?"

Nurse: "Yes! She is shouting and swearing at us, she has already hit one of the nurses, we can't get her undressed and she wants to go out and buy some cigarettes."

From this brief conversation it might be concluded that the old lady was confused, aggressive and, to say the least, difficult. There is no doubt that the nurse/patient relationship was under considerable strain. Fortunately for all concerned, the resident on his way to the ward met the consultant who asked if Mrs Harris had yet been admitted. He went on to explain that she had come in for investigation of her anaemia which had not responded to treatment with oral iron. Since she was 85 it had been decided, in consultation with her general practitioner (GP), to bring her in to hospital, and as he knew there was a bed available he had arranged it with the ward. He added that one of the reasons underlying his action was that she was a strong-willed, dominant old lady who smoked like a chimney, ruled her family with a rod of iron and was impatient with inaction and inefficiency! On hearing the resident's story he laughed and said, "Well, has she got any cigarettes because she certainly won't settle down without them—maybe she genuinely wants to go out and buy some." They went together to the ward and sure enough this was the explanation for the old lady's apparently outrageous and confused behaviour. The doctor/patient relationship was therefore excellent, right from the begining though it took a little longer to restore the nurse/patient relationship! However, it should be recognised that had the nursing staff been told when the admission was arranged about her addiction to cigarettes the whole misunderstanding and episode might have been avoided. It is very important for all those who are involved in the management of the elderly patient to have as much information as possible about the subject in question. This applies just as much to those involved in the care of the patient at home, as it does to the patient in hospital.

As people age there is a tendency for them to become more rigid in their response to life and more set in their ways. Consequently simple routines become much more important and their omission or alteration can give rise to frustration, and sometimes confusion. Decision-making may also become more difficult and routine hospital administrative procedures prove obstacles to treatment; for example, signing an anaesthetic consent form may take time because of the need for reassurance and explanation; or moving the position of his bed may make a patient confused. As will be seen later (Chapter 9), there is often a subtle deterioration in memory with age, short-term memory and ability to recall things to order being particularly affected. History taking, therefore, becomes more difficult and time consuming than in the young. While cues may help the old person to remember they can also trigger inappropriate responses and lead the questioner away from the point!

PROBLEMS OF COMMUNICATION

These relate primarily to speech and hearing, though lack of understanding may also play its part. Age changes in the vocal cords and larynx can alter the timbre of the voice and diminution of its force may make speech difficult to hear. Similarly lesions affecting the mouth and teeth, particularly ill-fitting false teeth, may also have effects, which may be remediable. Vision may also play a part in identifying cues, following gestures in attracting attention and understanding written material. Neurological disease is common in old age and aphasia and dysarthria are often complications. The advice of a speech therapist should be sought as soon as possible with regard to both conditions, because the assessment of the speech deficit is important and may be helped by aids such as pictures.

Deafness is frequently denied by old people, but they will admit to being hard of hearing and they can often hear well if speech is clearly, slowly and loudly enunciated. Shouting is not only embarrassing, but often unnecessary and may be painful to the patient (Chapter 6). When speaking to a deaf person it is important to position yourself so that your face is seen clearly, for many old people have considerable lip reading ability. Deafness is often due to the accumulation of wax in the ears, though removal of the wax may not be possible at the time of the initial examination and a detailed history may have to wait until this has been done. Hearing aids can be of considerable value in establishing easy communication. The speaking tube or ear trumpet is one type of hearing aid which is of great value in the outpatient clinic or surgery or the patient's home. It amplifies without distorting sound, is cheap and should be part of the equipment of every doctor, nurse and social worker who has regular contact with old people. A more sophisticated electronic communicator is also extremely effective, is relatively inexpensive and should be available both in geriatric wards and day hospitals.

SPECIAL POINTS TO ELICIT FROM THE OLDER PATIENT

One feature which often distinguishes the elderly patient from others is a limited capacity for self-care. Old people often depend on the help of others to maintain their place in the community. This dependence may be due to old age alone or, more likely, to old age linked to disability resulting from a pathological process. The capacity to deal with a personal environment is of great importance. To quote a simple example, someone who is unable to climb stairs on account of breathlessness will be totally marooned if he lives in a second-floor flat that has no lift, but might be independent if he lived in a bungalow or ground-floor flat in an area with level surroundings. It is essential that information relating to the home environment is included in the clinical record, for this knowledge will aid the overall management plan and facilitate early discharge.

The patient's outlook on his own ability must be checked with the insights of others (Chapter 9); these may include the GP, district nurse, health visitor, other professional observers or relatives, friends, and neighbours. It is quite common for different people to vary in their opinion of an individual's ability and the type of provision needed for future care. A detailed social history which clearly states and distinguishes the view of the patient from others who have been concerned with his care in the community is of vital importance in reaching a rational and agreed decision about further management. It is, however, essential that the assessment is as unbiased as possible, and account taken of the possible prejudices of those consulted. The patient's wishes should be taken into consideration and, if realistic, met. Carers, though, may need counselling and given relief as required. Such a planned procedure saves a lot of time and is likely to solve the problem which most concerns the patient. Many of the more esoteric medical and social conditions which the professional worker uncovers may be of little importance.

SOCIAL ACCEPTABILITY(Cases 4 and 8)

A patient's history must record details of behaviour and habits, because the ease or difficulty of the discharge will often depend on whether these are acceptable to others. While this information may be discovered by direct questioning of the patient, it is more likely to be obtained from those who have known him for a long time at home. The most striking example of a behavioural problem is incontinence, obviously a social barrier as well as an unpleasant state for the patient, yet likely to be concealed because of the social stigma attached to the condition (Chapter 14).

NUTRITION

The subject of nutrition is discussed in Chapter 6. A detailed history is often difficult to obtain from the patient, but it should be attempted and checked with relatives whenever sub-nutrition or over-nutrition is suspected.

PHYSICAL EXAMINATION

Physical examination of the elderly patient varies little from that of the younger patient. One or two special points are worth noting in each system.

General. The general appearance in relation to age is often helpful. The youthful-looking "old old" person usually has less underlying pathological change.

Cyanosis, malar flush and coldness of the extremities may indicate a low tissue oxygen saturation resulting from a low cardiac output.

An assessment of nutritional state and hydration should be noted, particularly when loss of weight or wasting are present. During the examination it is important to continue talking to the patient—it is reassuring and courteous and also provides further invaluable and confirmatory history. Similarly, the patient's mood, appropriateness of response, etc., can all be assessed and recorded during physical examination.

Cardiovascular system. The apex beat is often difficult to feel, as are the pulses in the legs and feet; nevertheless, it is important to record the presence or absence of all peripheral pulses as well as the state of the arterial wall. It is often advantageous, if feasible, to examine the patient after exercise if that is a stimulus to symptoms. Blood pressure should always be recorded supine and erect.

Respiratory system. Age changes in lung tissue as well as weakness of the accessory muscles of respiration mean that physical signs may be less evident. The most useful sign indicating lung disease is an increase in the respiratory rate, rising to 28/min or more. This sign may precede radiological lung changes (Chapter 11).

Central nervous system. The fundi may be difficult to see and the pupils may require dilatation; a good ophthalmoscope is needed and the doctor should be competent in its use. Ankle jerks are often absent, but this is not necessarily an indication of pathological change. Absent vibration sense in the legs is common but may not indicate disease. When possible, the patient should be asked to stand and walk so that his balance and gait can be assessed. Minor motor, coordination and sensory disturbances often only become apparent when this is done.

Endocrine. Small goitres are often present and are easily missed. The testes are often smaller and harder than normal. Loss of hair is evident over the body but is not associated with gross endocrine changes. Baldness is common and may be embarrassing to women.

Alimentary system. The dental state and whether or not dentures are worn should always be recorded.

Physical signs of the acute abdomen are often hard to elicit. The absence of bowel sounds may be the only indication that something is amiss.

Locomotor system. Abnormalities are common and may limit mobility. The state of the feet should always be recorded; abnormalities are common and are frequently remediable thereby improving mobility. An opportunity should be taken to observe the patient getting out of a chair or bed and during walking whenever possible. This often reveals that the locomotor problem is due to pain, weakness, stiffness or instability.

Skin. The state of the skin should be noted. Skinfold thickness diminishes with age but most of the changes attributed to age (wrinkles, sallowness, bagginess) are more likely the effect of over-exposure to ultraviolet light. This also leads to malignant changes in the skin such as solar keratoses, basal cell carcinoma (rodent ulcer) and squamous cell carcinoma. Skin lesions may also indicate underlying visceral neoplasms either by the occurrence of skin metastases or other change in the skin such as the flexural pigmentation seen in acanthosis nigricans. Similarly other changes, such as the mottled pigmented lesion of the lower limbs, erythema ab igne, common in old ladies who sit too close to the fire in winter, may indicate poor circulation in the legs or even hypothyroidism. Very thin skin of the back of the hands may indicate a similar state in the bones.

Immune system. Ageing is associated with a deterioration in the immediate and delayed response of the immune system to injury or infection. This state is further accentuated by poor nutrition, and chronic conditions such as chronic renal failure, non-insulin dependent diabetes mellitus and rheumatoid arthritis. Practical implications of this are that signs and symptoms of acute illness are often masked. In bronchopneumonia, for example, no pyrexia may occur, there is little change in the leucocyte count and the localising signs in the chest are minimal (Chapter 11). Similarly in tuberculosis an impaired immunological response may prevent a diagnostic response to the intradermal injection of tuberculin.

THE PROBLEM LIST (see cases)

The use of problem-orientated medical records in the care of the elderly is invaluable and enables a continuing review of the individual's problems to be made. However, it must be stressed that building up the whole picture from a history and examination of the elderly patient takes time. It is probably best to start by listing the major presenting problem or problems and then adding to these as more information becomes available. Once a list has been made a plan of action can be prepared for each specific problem. Initially, this may indicate the need for much more information which, in turn, may lead to the addition of further problems to the initial list. Almost certainly then this list will need sorting out. This can be done at a case conference (Chapter 5), when the health team together with patient and those supporting him/her at home can prioritise the problems to be tackled with the objective of making him/her as independent as possible.

FURTHER READING

Gravell, R. (1988). *Communication Problems in Elderly People*. London: Croom Helm.

Horwitz, A., Macfadyen, D.M., Scrimshaw, N.S. *et al.* (1989). *Nutrition in the Elderly*. Oxford: Oxford University Press.

Monk, B.E., Graham-Brown, R.A.C. and Sarkany, I. (1988). *Skin Disorders in the Elderly*. Oxford: Blackwell Scientific.

Seymour, G. (1986). *Medical Assessment of the Elderly Surgical Patient*. London: Croom Helm.

Stuart-Hamilton, I. (1991). *The Psychology of Ageing*. London: Jessica Kingsley.

CHAPTER 3 Clinical investigation in the elderly

It is well recognised that the elderly suffer from more than one disease process at a time and that if a patient is to be treated correctly the diagnosis must be as precise as possible. The doctor must find out not only what is troubling the patient most, but when clinical problems may underlie his complaint and whether it is possible to put these right. Having talked to the patient, his relatives and others closest to him about his problems (if he has no objection to this) and having examined him to assess mental and physical capacity we may now direct attention to the function of individual organs. This may involve chemical analysis of the blood, urine, faeces or sputum, and X-rays may need to be taken of bones, soft tissues and internal organs. Electrical tracings of heart and brain function, ultrasound recordings of the abdomen, computed tomography, and biopsies of skin, bone marrow or internal organs also may be necessary. The problems, therefore, that face the clinical investigator are firstly, how much investigation is justified, secondly how valuable are the tests and, thirdly, where should they be done?

HOW MUCH INVESTIGATION IS JUSTIFIED?

Sometimes this can be a difficult question to answer. The prime consideration must be the overall benefit that will accrue to the patient. It has been pointed out already that it is common for several disease processes to coexist in the same patient. One of the commonest ways for illness to present in the elderly is "failure to thrive". In other words, the patient presents with symptoms of being unwell and further enquiry may only elicit an indeterminate symptom such as tiredness or generalised weakness, so that finding a cause is often time consuming and difficult. Hence, it is easier for the physician to ascribe the symptom to old age rather than to a disease, or to prescribe a non-specific treatment in the hope that the symptom will go away. The treatment given will often depend on the physician's whim or whatever fashion is in current vogue: Substances frequently prescribed are iron, vitamins, tranquillisers, antidepressants, other types of "happy pills", anabolic steroids, "cerebral activators", and other substances, sometimes classified under the heading of "geripeutics"! The only beneficial effect of many of these will be that of a placebo, while some will do more harm than good. Fortunately in recent years the action of the Committee for Review of Medicines has removed many of these substances from the National Formulary so that they no longer are available.

If the purpose of the investigation is explained, the patient will usually cooperate fully (Chapter 2, "The elderly patient as an individual"). It must be remembered that any investigation can be construed as an "assault". It is most important therefore that the patient gives "informed consent" to the procedures which are to be used. The objective of any investigation is to aid the long- and short-term management plan of the person in question. It should also be recognised that extensive investigation of multiple pathology is likely to cause considerable distress, discomfort and inconvenience. The reason for initiating any investigation must be clear, and no "routine" investigation should ever be performed unless it can be justified in terms of benefit to the patient or to others who might be in contact.

Age, *per se*, only rarely should be a bar to investigation. The condition of the subject and the potential quality of his future life are the prime considerations. A demented centenarian with clinical evidence of heart failure and bronchopneumonia obviously does not require any investigation, unless there is a potential risk to the nursing staff involved. If for example, there was a past history of tuberculosis, sputum examination and culture would be necessary. A centenarian who, until the current illness, had been fairly independent, i.e. one of the "young old" (Chapter 1), is another matter, particularly if the underlying condition is likely to respond to treatment, thereby enabling a return home to an active life, or one which the individual considers acceptable. Investigation might involve radiological procedures, including contrast studies, ultrasonography, and endoscopy in addition to haematological and biochemical analysis of blood. Wherever possible, tests used to investigate any older patient should be non-invasive. All should relate to the patient's health in terms of comfortable survival and it may be better to obtain a specialist opinion before resorting to a battery of uncomfortable and potentially hazardous tests. Radiologists, for example, now have considerable experience in investigating older patients and joint discussion and consultation of selected patients can be invaluable, for not only will the patient meet the doctor who will be performing the investigation but the procedure will be explained with greater accuracy.

HOW VALUABLE ARE THE TESTS?

A "valuable" test is one which will give a high return in terms of treatable disease, or indicates the need for further, more extensive investigation. If the latter, then further consideration can be given as to whether such investigation is justifiable and acceptable to the patient and where it should be undertaken. From the patient's point of view a "valuable" test is one which causes him the least possible inconvenience and disruption to his life. Consequently blood tests or simple biopsies, which can be undertaken in the GP's surgery or even in the patient's own home, are more acceptable than tests which need a visit to hospital, which, in turn, are more acceptable than tests that require a stay in hospital.

A "valuable" test is also one that gives an unequivocal result that enables firm decisions to be taken. Unfortunately, it is almost universal that variation in physiological and other individual parameters increases with increasing age. Whether this is due to the "ageing process" or latent disease is often not known. Consequently what is "normal" for one person may not be so for another. It is possible that the definition of much narrower "normal ranges" in old age may result from analysis of longitudinal studies currently being undertaken in Sweden and in the United States of America. At the present time, comparison with results of similar tests recorded in the patient's own past medical record may be the only indicator of abnormality.

Haematological Tests (Cases 4 and 10)

Most of the standard haematological indices are unaffected by age so that the same values can be placed on these tests as in younger people. The incidence of anaemia, however, increases with age so that haematological investigation will tend to give a fairly high return in terms of treatable disease (Chapter 12).

The white cell count tends to fall with age due to a lower proportion of lymphocytes: the range is usually given as from 3×10^9 to 9×10^9/l. Levels in the upper normal range or just above should be viewed with suspicion for they may indicate a granulocytic response to infection.

The erythrocyte sedimentation rate (ESR) tends to rise with age being slightly higher in women than in men, though it is likely that population studies have included some abnormal subjects. Consequently the value of this test as a discriminator between health and disease is less in the older subject. Nevertheless very high levels of around 100 mm/h should not be disregarded and levels over 30 mm/h should be viewed with suspicion and the subject examined carefully.

Biochemical Tests (Cases 2 and 7)

Many of the biochemical values which are accepted as normal in younger patients also apply to the elderly. The ability of the kidney to excrete nitrogenous waste products may be impaired in some elderly so that their blood urea may be slightly elevated, a level of up to 10 mmol/l being accepted as normal compared with a range of from 2.5 to 6.6 mmol/l in younger individuals (Chapter 13, "renal function"): this is due to a reduced glomerular filtration rate. This observation is important because if the renal reserve is reduced the blood urea is likely to rise to even higher levels in situations of stress. Hence patients with acute infection such as pneumonia might have blood urea levels of 15–20 mmol/l (Case 2). Such levels are usually indicative of renal failure in a younger patient but this may not apply in the elderly. Similarly, serum creatinine has a higher upper limit in old age, as does the serum uric acid. The diagnosis of renal failure is, therefore, more difficult and high uric acid levels do not always diagnose gout. Paradoxically, it is not unusual to find patients with creatinine levels below 130 μmol/l who have an abnormally low creatinine clearance. This may be explained by a low rate of production secondary to a reduced lean body mass (Chapters 7 and 13).

High serum calcium concentrations are often found coincidentally in old people. More common causes for this include primary hyperparathyroidism, skeletal metastases, multiple myeloma and vitamin D intoxication. If no clinical symptoms are associated with the hypercalcaemia due to hyperparathyroidism, this is best left untreated (Chapter 7). Low levels of serum calcium may also be found; this may indicate osteomalacia, a relatively common condition in elderly housebound women living in northern climes (Chapter 7). Since a low calcium level may also be due to low levels of albumin, most laboratories use a simple formula which "corrects" the serum calcium concentration for albumin levels. This is important for ill health and subnutrition in old age often leads to low albumin levels.

Some old people have low serum potassium levels. While diuretic therapy is a cause, a deficient dietary intake of potassium is common. Minor degrees of diarrhoea, often due to excess laxative use, also will lead to increased potassium loss. Though the serum potassium bears little relationship to total body stores, it is a useful test nevertheless, since it is the potassium serum level rather than the cellular level, which determines most of the symptoms. These include myocardial excitability, muscle weakness and gut atony. Low magnesium levels may be more common than is generally realised and in one study one-third of the patients attending a geriatric day hospital had low levels. Many of these had low calcium levels and the serum calcium rose when magnesium was given in small doses by mouth. By far the commonest cause of magnesium deficiency was diuretic therapy. The deficiency also causes hypokalaemia (low serum potassium), which is resistant to potassium supplementation unless magnesium is also given.

As has been indicated already, the serum levels of various biochemical indices are affected by disease processes and their treatment. As with albumin, similar changes affect other carrier proteins such as thyroxine binding globulin and iron binding protein and we need to make appropriate allowance for this, in the same way as we do for calcium. Similarly, as with potassium, other electrolytes such as sodium are affected and hyponatraemia (low serum sodium) is frequently seen in acutely ill patients admitted to the acute geriatric ward. These factors must be remembered when planning treatment, particularly when many patients admitted with acute illness are also dehydrated (Chapter 13).

Endocrine Tests (Case 6)

Because diabetes mellitus and disorders of the thyroid gland are common in old age, blood sugar estimations and tests of thyroid function may be of considerable value in diagnosing these conditions, as they are in the younger patient. However, as indicated above, the effects of age and illness need to be taken into account when assessing the results. Other endocrine disorders do occur in old people but the tests required for their diagnosis are similar to those used in younger patients and the "normal ranges" are unchanged.

Diabetes mellitus (Chapter 13)

The renal threshold for glucose rises with age; as a result testing the urine for sugar may not be as reliable as in the younger patient. The most useful test to do if the diagnosis is suspected is a fasting venous blood glucose. The normal fasting plasma glucose level should be below 8.0 mmol/l (144 mg/dl); if not the patient is diabetic. If doubt remains a glucose tolerance test should be done. A standard 75 g glucose challenge was introduced by the National Diabetes Data Group in 1979. The recommendations made with regard to "normal" criteria for the test require minor modification in the older patient. It has been suggested that observations should be continued for 3 hours since the rate of fall in the plasma glucose level may be important, a fall of 2.8 mmol/l (50 mg/dl) or more from 1 to 3 hours indicating normal glucose homeostasis. Upper limits of 13.3 mmol/l (240 mg/dl) at 1 hour, 12.2 mmol/l (220mg/dl) at 2 hours and 10.6 mmol/l (190 mg/dl) at 3 hours have been suggested as reasonable since they may prevent an inappropriate diagnosis of glucose intolerance being made.

Thyroid disease (Cases 5 and 6)

The incidence of both overactivity (hyperthyroidism) and underactivity (hypothyroidism) (Chapter 13) is of the order of 1 to 3% in patients admitted to geriatric units. However, as has already been pointed out, alteration in the levels of carrier proteins associated with acute illness and its drug treatment may affect tests of thyroid function. Consequently, evaluation of the various tests available must take into account the numerous factors which can give rise to misleading results. Most laboratories measure thyroid-stimulating hormone (TSH) as a screening test for thyroid disease. High levels (>4.0 mU/l) indicating hypothyroidism and low levels (<0.2 mU/l) indicating hyperthyroidism. If the TSH is borderline, free or total thyroxine (T_4) levels should be measured. If doubts as to the diagnosis still remain, and the effects of illness and drugs have been taken into account, then the response of the pituitary and thyroid glands to an injection of thyrotrophin-releasing hormone (TRH) can be measured. This is particularly useful in diagnosing doubtful cases of hypothyroidism where the basal TSH level is only minimally raised, as patients with this condition show an exaggerated and prolonged TSH response to TRH.

Anti-thyroid antibodies are commonly raised in older people, particularly women. High titres may be associated with thyroid disease and thyroid function tests should be performed in such patients. The value of this test is probably low, except possibly for population screening.

Radiological Investigation (Cases 2, 5, 6, 9 and 10)

Apart from simple radiological investigations, such as a posteroanterior (PA) chest and straight X-ray of the abdomen, it is probably wise to consult with the radiologist when more extensive procedures may be indicated. No X-ray should be ordered as a routine procedure, since this wastes valuable time and money. The two X-rays mentioned are the most useful simple ones to request. The chest X-ray gives information on the state of the lungs (Chapter 11) and heart size (Chapter 10), and also gives information on the state of the skeleton, being helpful in assessing the degree of osteoporosis or osteomalacia (Chapter 7). An abdominal X-ray should be taken to include both hip joints. It will then not only show the faecal content of the bowel but also possible skeletal and joint disease. Other changes, including aortic and vascular calcification, may be seen as well as gallstones and soft tissue shadows of kidneys and bladder.

Ultrasonography is being used increasingly for the investigation of intra-abdominal conditions. It is of value in the assessment of renal masses, liver secondaries and gallstones, prostatic disease and other pelvic disease (particularly as an aid to accurate biopsy). Increasing use has led to increased skill in the use and therefore value of the investigation. Moreover, being relatively non-invasive it is acceptable to elderly patients, although explanation of the procedure is still essential to allay anxiety.

Computed tomography (CT) of the brain (Case 9) and whole body is now widely available. Its use may be of great value in planning the long- and short-term management of the patient for it can make accurate diagnosis possible and hence save time and money. Recent developments of this technique such as positron emission tomography (PET) and nuclear magnetic resonance imaging (MRI) enable tissues to be scanned and organs, such as the brain, mapped so that lesions may be accurately localised. These advances will undoubtedly benefit the elderly and the tests should be used whenever they are likely to modify management. PET scanning and MR spectroscopy also are valuable as research tools to study brain function in normal and abnormal ageing.

Echocardiography

Recent developments in the three types of echocardiography (M-mode, cross-sectional and Doppler) allow non-invasive assessment of cardiac form and function and consequently the diagnosis of cardiac disease. This is essential for the accurate assessment of cardiac failure (diastolic versus systolic function), the severity of valvular disease and the diagnosis of subacute bacterial endocarditis. It is, therefore, very helpful in the selection of suitable patients for cardiac surgery, and in identifying those in whom treatment with angiotensin-converting enzymes (ACE) inhibitors would be inappropriate (Chapter 10).

Urinalysis

Urinalysis still has a part to play in the assessment of the elderly patient, although it is not as important as in a younger patient. Microscopy and culture are valuable in that large numbers of pus cells usually indicate infection and culture establishes the offending organism enabling treatment to be effective. Haematuria, even if only microscopic, warrants investigation at any age. Chemical analysis is less valuable. Though elderly patients with micro-albuminuria have a reduced life expectancy, this information is of limited value in the practical management of individual patients. Similarly, as mentioned earlier, glycosuria may be absent even when the patient has diabetes (Chapter 13).

Bacteriological Investigation

Bacteriological investigation of various body fluids is very helpful in the management and treatment of the elderly patient. It is difficult, sometimes, to get uncontaminated specimens of some fluids. Urine particularly presents problems (Chapter 14). Nevertheless, examination and culture of sputum or pus from a joint effusion or other serous cavity may be a life-saving procedure by indicating the most effective antibiotic to be used. Blood cultures themselves may be especially helpful in confirming the presence of an infective organism and its sensitivity to antibiotics. The normal immune response may be compromised by disease and poor nutrition so that pyrexia and other signs of infection may be absent in the early stages of septicaemia, and resort to early blood culture may be the only chance of saving the patient's life. Indeed in such cases sending blood for bacteriological examination and culture needs to be the first investigation undertaken.

OTHER INVESTIGATIONS

All the usual investigations such as electroencephalography, electrocardiography, electromyography, radio-isotope scanning, endoscopy, bronchoscopy (Case 9) and biopsies of bone, muscle, skin, artery and other organs and tissues may be of value in determining the management of selected patients. Further comment on some of these is necessary.

Electroencephalography (EEG)

With the advent of CT, MRI and PET scanning the value of the EEG has diminished as a diagnostic tool in old age. It may be helpful still in the diagnosis of variable or episodic behavioural abnormalities. An example is that epilepsy may present in bizarre ways and the EEG may be useful as an initial screening test (Chapter 8).

Electrocardiography (ECG)

Tracings are frequently abnormal and community surveys have shown that about half the elderly have some alteration of wave

form. Many of these are insignificant or, at least, require no therapeutic action. The ECG is most useful in the diagnosis of arrhythmias and in determining digitalis toxicity (Case 7), which is often
associated with low potassium levels (hypokalaemia). Continuous
ambulatory telemetric ECG monitoring may be particularly useful
in diagnosing dysrhythmias (Case 5), which are often transient
and are associated with "dizzy" spells, falls and other transitory
symptoms (Chapters 8 and 10). However, transient arrhythmias
are common even in healthy old people, and only are significant
if they can be linked to symptoms. This can be difficult in frail
patients with limited compliance.

Endoscopy (Cases 4 and 10)

Endoscopy as a special investigation now presents a major advance
in the management of the elderly patient. If one includes laparo-
scopy as an endoscopic procedure there is almost no part of the
body that cannot be examined by direct vision through some form
of optical instrument! The urologist has pioneered the use of the
endoscope to study the bladder and lower urinary tract and developed the technique so that transurethral resection of the prostate
has become the treatment of choice for urinary tract obstruction
due to prostatic hypertrophy. The gastroenterologist has followed
suit with endoscopic examination of the upper and lower gastrointestinal tract thereby improving diagnosis, as well as treatment,
particularly of peptic ulcer. Recent developments have enabled the
investigation of the pancreatic and common bile ducts and the
removal of calculi from the latter (Chapter 12). The elderly seem
to tolerate endoscopy extremely well and the sedation given seems
to remove all memory of the procedure. In many, the procedure
is preferred to a barium meal examination. There is no doubt that
these advances hold considerable promise and many frail elderly
may be able to receive treatment that was formerly denied to them.
Nevertheless although such treatment is relatively non-invasive, it
should not be undertaken lightly and only then after full explanation.

WHERE SHOULD INVESTIGATIONS BE DONE?

Earlier in this chapter we suggested that investigation should cause
as little disruption to the patient's life as possible. The aim, there-

fore, should be for as many investigations as possible to be done on an outpatient basis. It must be remembered that some investigations are tiring for frail or elderly patients and it may be necessary to investigate them at a day hospital or to use day beds in which they can recover. Under these circumstances someone must be at home to care for them when they return, for they may need support for a day or two. All investigations, therefore, should be planned and discussed with all concerned, if full value is to be obtained from them, and the elderly patient inconvenienced as little as possible.

The main purpose of investigation is to initiate treatment that will make the patient more comfortable and improve the quality of his life. Sometimes, though, investigation will show that treatment is unlikely to be effective even when the investigation was justifiable. Clinicians in other specialties may sometimes have difficulty in understanding the need for investigation (or for that matter treatment) without prior consultation and explanation. Such consultation should not be forgotten, for only by such interdisciplinary consultation and cooperation will those practising medicine in the elderly become acquainted with "senile" pathology and surmount its difficulties.

FURTHER READING

Beech, J.R. and Harding, L. (1990). *Assessment of the Elderly.* Windsor: NFER-Nelson.

Hodkinson, H.M. (1984). *Clinical Biochemistry of the Elderly.* London: Churchill Livingstone.

MacLennan, W.J. and Peden, N.R. (1989). *Metabolic and Endocrine Problems in the Elderly.* London: Springer Verlag.

CHAPTER 4 Social problems and the elderly

INTRODUCTION

Definition. "A social problem may be defined as arising when the continuing placement of an individual in the community causes social stress, which is perceived to be unacceptable to those concerned with the care of the individual, or the individual himself and is not amenable to medical treatment".

The elderly patient is often termed a "social problem" by doctors. This is because they perceive the future management of the case as pertaining more to social care than to medical care. In other words the doctor, whether a GP or hospital specialist, feels that medical skill has no further part to play in the patient's illness, and that the patient only requires "looking after" by someone who will help him to perform the essential activities of daily living. In the case of the GP, the referral may be either to the local department of social services, or to the local health authority's geriatric (or psychogeriatric) service. In the case of the hospital specialist, the referral is often to the geriatric service or the social worker for "disposal", because attempts to discharge the patient have failed and it is considered that further treatment, in the specialist setting, will not improve the patient's performance. Modern organisation of hospital medical services has helped to avoid this sort of situation arising as frequently as it did, for in many hospitals geriatric medicine is integrated closely with acute services, so that management plans for patients who are likely to need some form of long-term or continuing care are made early in their admission. Alternatively, geriatric medicine may operate an age defined admission policy so that these patients are admitted direct to the service. Such organisation of services should help to prevent social stress for patients and their relatives and make the management of the "social problem" easier. Now that the GP is contracted to offer assessment to all his patients over 75 years, on a yearly basis, his knowledge of the older patient should already be greater. He should know the social state of individuals and be able to draft a provisional, long-term management plan. The management of these patients also may become even easier after April 1993 when the NHS and Community Care Act (1990) becomes law. Though responsibility for the continuing care of these elderly patients will be passed to the local authority (LA) social services department (SSD), the health authority (HA) will continue to retain responsibility for those, who require continuing nursing care. The HAs may contract this service out to geriatric or psychogeriatric units, to private care organisations or to private or voluntary nursing homes. Though a decision as to the most appropriate service may be made on the basis of cost, close collaboration will be needed between the HA and the SSD in order to define which authority will be responsible for care and who will pay. However, in the patient's interest, it is essential that "arms-length" inspection teams, who are independent of the statutory authorities, are appointed to ensure standards are maintained at a high level.

An important provision of the Community Care Act is that priority will be given to maintaining an elderly individual at home, or in "homely settings" in the community and that institutionalisation will only be considered if, even with maximum social and health care back-up, this is found to be impracticable. The professional responsible for organising community care will be a "care manager". His first task will be to arrange for a full medical and social assessment of the client by appropriate professionals. On the basis of this he will define the needs of the client and after consultation with the client and his carers (if any), will plan a package of care. The next step will be to commission appropriate services to provide this. Thereafter, it will be his duty, to evaluate the effectiveness of the package, and to review this regularly to determine continuing need.

It is likely that the professional background to the "care manager" will vary with the particular needs of the client. If the system is to work it is essential that the "care manager" has appropriate training, and is able to command the respect of other professionals. His task will not be an easy one, for past research has shown that the "professional" assessment of a client's need does not always agree with the client's own opinion nor that of a lay observer. It will also be essential that the SSD has adequate financial resources, to meet the heavy costs of providing adequate community care.

For severely incapacitated individuals, home care may be preferable to institutionalisation but, certainly, is not less expensive. It is unlikely that it will be possible to provide optimal care to all in need, and hence a system of priorities will have to be developed.

THE CAUSES OF SOCIAL PROBLEMS

Social stress sufficient to cause a social problem usually occurs because an individual has lost the ability to perform those activities of daily living necessary to live independently, without being a hazard or risk to himself and/or others. If "social" problems are considered as "performance" problems then their solution may be easier (see Figure 1.4). Their many causes may be listed as follows.

Physical Disability (Cases 5 and 8)

This is one of the commonest underlying causes. It is easy to understand why this should be, since disability, whether due to disease or age, sufficient to prevent an individual performing the normal everyday activities of daily living means that someone's help is needed. If no help is available and ability cannot be improved either by medical amelioration, rehabilitative measures or by altering living arrangements then the risk of hazards such as neglect and ill health increases and may impose a high level of stress on others. Physical disability resulting in functional deficiency has many causes. It is often attributed to "just old age" (Chapter 6); it may be associated with lesions of the musculoskeletal system (Chapter 7); or may be due to diseases of the neurological system, the commonest cause being "stroke" with associated paralysis (Chapter 8). Whatever the reason every effort must be made to maximise ability, and if this fails, the individual should be cared for in an environment of his choice (Case 5).

Mental Disability (Case 4)

This is another common cause of a social problem because of the stress it produces on carers. It may take the form of an acute illness (delirium), dementia, or an affective disorder, usually a depressive illness, or another psychiatric disorder. These conditions are discussed in Chapters 6 and 9 but one must go beyond the diagnosis to define the particular practical problems which are causing distress to the carer and try to find solutions. An example is that nocturnal restlessness may be extremely distressing, but may respond to a simple measure, such as a small blackboard placed where it is easily seen with the word "night" written on it, the patient being told that he must stay in bed until this reads "day".

Social Incompetence (Case 4)

This usually is the result of a physical or mental disease process, but there are also some people who are bad managers and always have been. Earlier in life, they may have been spoilt by an over-caring spouse, parent or sibling, so that they have never learned to cope with the more mundane routines of life, such as cooking meals, washing clothes, shopping, managing household accounts, etc. Such individuals may be intelligent and capable of learning, but some will always have had a learning difficulty and have been protected by their more able relatives. With age their limited intellectual ability will have diminished so that they require continuing support in a sheltered environment. It is most important to exclude disease, before putting people into this category or labelling them as demented.

Difficult Personalities (Cases 3 and 8)

It has been said that as people age they become caricatures of their previous personality. This can mean that their more unpleasant traits become accentuated and they become more difficult to live with. Such people may well give rise to social stress and consequently be referred as a social problem. They include: the strong-willed dominant person who will often accept neglect and discomfort as a reasonable price to pay for independence, insisting on living alone at home, yet needing considerable support which is often only grudgingly accepted; the chronic manipulator whose skill in using frailties, situations and human beings to his own advantage will sometimes drive relatives to suicide or assault (elder abuse); the frankly abnormal person who may lead the life of a recluse or present with "Diogenes syndrome", collecting large amounts of useless material such as newspapers, potato crisp packets, etc., and living in dirt and squalor. These latter people are often in social classes 1 and 2.

Antisocial Behaviour (Cases 2 and 8)

Aggression, noisiness, dirty habits (faecal smearing or hiding "parcels" of excreta in drawers, etc.), urinary incontinence, nocturnal wandering, inappropriate urination (e.g. into the fireplace), nakedness and exposure are all examples of behaviour which create stress in carers and others. Relief of carers before situations become unbearable must be initiated, urgently, if long-term institutional care is to be avoided. The underlying cause of the abnormal behaviour must be carefully assessed and, if possible, treated or remedied. It must be remembered that antisocial behaviour, occasionally, can be a gesture of anger or a protest against the situation in which the individual finds himself. For instance, a 92-year-old man was referred on account of antisocial behaviour, in this case inappropriate micturition over his daughter-in-law's lounge carpet. It transpired that he liked to go out to the pub and being unsteady on his feet, tended to stagger. This embarrassed her for "what would the neighbours think", so she kept him a virtual prisoner in a sparsely furnished room. That social problem was solved by restoring the old man's freedom!

ATTITUDES IN RELATION TO SOCIAL PROBLEMS
(Cases 2, 4, 5, 8, and 9)

The Social Worker

The main need of the elderly client is to be able to express his perceived need to someone who will listen sympathetically and then do something about it. That person is often the social worker, who must assess what it is that the client wants and, after discussion, organise resources to meet that need. Frequently the social worker may be the first point of contact in the assessment of the elderly client. He, therefore, must have knowledge of the ageing process and the diseases and disabilities which afflict old people. He needs to be able to collaborate with and relate to health professionals who may be treating the elderly person, as well as the relatives and others concerned with their management. It is essential, for the proper assessment of need, that the social worker has access to all the information that is available about the client. A good computerised, information system is necessary to achieve this. This will become even more important after April 1993 when the NHS and Community Care Act becomes effective and many social workers will be "care managers", responsible for purchasing the resources necessary to maintain the client at home, for as long as possible. In this situation the social worker will need to know all the resources that exist to support the individual, their availability, their cost, the circumstances in which they are likely to be effective and their degree of substitutability, so that they may be used in the most cost-effective manner.

When confronted with a client's problem, the social worker has to decide what is the most reasonable solution and this will only be achieved if the social worker's attitude is that of a friend and arbiter to the client. The wishes of the client are paramount even when they seem unrealistic and impracticable. If sufficiently motivated, old people sometimes can overcome great disability and handicap and continue to live in their own homes despite the opposition of relatives, friends and neighbours, and health care professionals.

It is not uncommon, when such strong-willed people refuse to do what others would wish of them and insist on their human rights, that the judgement of the social worker is called into question by the relatives and others. In these circumstances the social worker's role is unenviable. Nevertheless, if the wishes of the elderly client are to be fulfilled, and it is clear that the individual concerned is in full possession of his mental faculties, it is vital that the social worker displays tact and patience while allowing relatives and others to work through their fears and anxieties. The resolution of such cases to the client's satisfaction, and with the eventual acceptance by the relatives and others that this was the right solution, can give the social worker great work satisfaction.

Health Professionals

Doctors are not the only health professionals to have varying attitudes to the "social problem"; nurses, medical students and other workers may be as bad. Attitudes, though, have improved considerably since this book was first written. This is undoubtedly due to the much greater volume of teaching given to all those involved in the NHS both pre- and post-qualification. However, a few remain who will still label, the patient as a "social problem", ignoring the underlying physical and/or mental disorders. This usually happens as a result of pressure, in the case of the primary health team worker, from relatives or other carers suffering from the social stress imposed on them; or in the case of the hospital staff, in the casualty department when it is extremely busy late on a Friday or Saturday night. Then, a frail old lady, living alone, subject to frequent falls, "sent-in" by the neighbours as an emergency by ambulance will be admitted reluctantly as a "social admission". Whereas in the past she remained labelled as a "social problem", now, she is more likely to be seen by someone from the geriatric service and the underlying cause of her recurrent falls investigated and treated, thereby curing her social problem.

Relatives, Friends and Neighbours (Cases 3, 4, 5 and 8)

The majority of disabled elderly people living at home are cared for by such "carers". Their time is given freely because of a sense of duty and compassion for another human being. In recent years their value has been recognised and "caring for carers" has become a need that must be met if the elderly person's wish to stay at home is to be granted. The "carer", therefore, must be given support and help to continue caring. It is easy to understand the anxieties and pressures which can be placed on "carers" when an elderly person becomes dependent on their help for their continuing survival in the community. This may happen gradually and be attributed to "old age" (Chapter 6), and in these cases "carers" may not notice the burden of care, and not seek help until they are at the end of their tether. In other cases dependency may occur suddenly after a fracture following a fall or as the result of a stroke. In these cases, help may be organised for the "carer" at an early stage. Support of the "carer" by the health professional is most important. It has been shown that professionals need to:

1. Respond to requests and arrange interviews promptly.
2. Make it clear who they are, where they have come from and why they have come.
3. Show sensitivity in their contact with the elderly individual.
4. Listen to the "carer" and be concerned about his well-being.
5. Give explanations that are clear and understandable.

6. Understand the possible reasons for confusion.
7. When dementia is diagnosed, establish the precise problems posed by its management, through careful questioning.
8. Agree with the "carer" a clear plan of action which is promptly implemented.
9. Respond immediately to "cries for help".

Given such adequate support nearly all carers will continue to look after their elderly dependent relatives and friends. However, in some cases, individuals may be a health hazard to others or require so much attention that continuing care at home is impossible. Then, the case may be brought to the notice of a magistrate who on the advice of two doctors may order admission to hospital for a period of 21 days, under Section 47 of the National Assistance Act (1947). Alternatively, a guardianship order may be made under Section 7 of the Mental Health Act (1983). To obtain the order application has to be made to the LA and be supported by two doctors and a qualified social worker or the nearest relative. The guardian will be either the SSD or a person accepted by them. In practice these procedures are rarely implemented. Most professionals and magistrates err on the side of freedom of choice by the patient and only overrule this in exceptional circumstances.

Financial Aspects

The basis for a social problem is often associated with poverty and lack of knowledge of statutory allowances that may be claimed. One of the major complaints that people have on retirement is shortage of money. In 1986 two-thirds of pensioners had incomes of less than 140% of the income support level. In 1988 a survey showed that 53% of elderly households had incomes of less than £100 a week, while only 18% had incomes of more than £200 a week. Moreover, elderly household incomes were lower in the over 75s. Similarly 62% had less than £2000 capital and only 18% had over £10 000. There is no doubt, therefore, that there are a lot of old people with little income and capital. It is desirable that all should have an income substantially above subsistence level.

As well as the basic pension most people will have an additional pension and a graduated pension, the three elements comprising the State Retirement Pension. Depending on the level of any occupational pension, income from savings and capital, additional benefits, such as income support, housing benefit, and relief from community charge, can all be claimed. Elderly people with disabilities may be eligible for additional benefits.

1. Attendance Allowance (two rates), which can be claimed by individuals requiring frequent attention or continual supervision after the day and/or night conditions have been fulfilled for 6 months. This period may be waived in the case of people who are terminally ill. It is not affected by income or savings and does not depend on National Insurance (NI) contributions. It is not taxable but has to be claimed by the person requiring help, who will be assessed by a visiting doctor.
2. Invalid Care Allowance, which can be claimed by the carer who is over 16 years and under pension age and spends a minimum of 35 hours a week looking after someone in receipt of attendance allowance. It is taxable.
3. Mobility Allowance which can be claimed by people who cannot walk or can only walk with great difficulty. Claims, however, must be made before the 66th birthday and the allowance will be paid until the age of 80 years or as long as the qualifying conditions are fulfilled. It can be paid to people at home or in hospital or another institution.
4. Monetary help may be obtainable for a variety of other things such as fuel, house insulation, repairs to property, paying for residential or nursing home care, and health costs not provided by the NHS.
5. Travel concessions are available on rail, underground, bus services and some airlines to pensioners.

While some of these pensions and benefits are available to all people who have reached retirement age and are qualified, others are means tested.

PRE-RETIREMENT EDUCATION

Most people who retire between the ages of 60 and 65 years have another 15 to 20 years of life ahead of them. Retirement must not be allowed to become an eventless interregnum between work and death. It must be recognised as a time of opportunity to make an increased contribution to society and a time for self-fulfilment and happiness. To achieve this, retirement must be planned. The basic requirements are health and money, which if possessed, will enable the individual to engage in recreational and leisure pursuits or participate in the activities of the voluntary services and remain amongst the young old.

Education about the ageing process and the problems of life after retirement should form part of all educational programmes. It is probably never too early to start and certainly some form of education concerning ageing and the ageing process should be undertaken prior to leaving school. Advice on pensions and savings needs to be given early in life and this applies to both sexes. In May 1990 the European Court of Justice ruled that men and women should be able to draw pension from the same age. An occupational pension in addition to the state pension is the most certain way of ensuring that an income in retirement is "substantially above subsistence level". If it is impossible to get into an occupational pension scheme then an insurance company must be approached and a personal scheme devised. Under the Social Security Act 1990 pension funds will have to guarantee minimal annual increases—limited price indexation (LPI). The Occupational Pensions Advisory Service (OPAS) was set up as a charity in 1982 and recently received a grant for the first time. OPAS works with the Citizens Advice Bureaux to help pensioners with queries. A pensions ombudsman was appointed in April 1990 to deal with tricky cases, which OPAS has not resolved. The pension scheme registry, once established, will be very useful in helping pensioners who have changed their jobs several times during their working life to trace the amounts and claim their dues. Hopefully, this better organisation of the general pension scene will eliminate the need for older people *having* to work in order to maintain their standard of living. The work ethic, though, will continue to operate in some individuals who should not be denied the right to work if they still wish to do so and can find work.

PRE-RETIREMENT AND POST-RETIREMENT COURSES

In many parts of the world, and in the United Kingdom in particular, such courses are organised. In the United Kingdom they may be run by a variety of organisations ranging from Universities to groups like the Workers Education Association or large employers who may organise their own courses. They make take the form of residential weekend courses, day-release courses or evening courses focusing on the various problems which the individual may face in retirement, and provide advice on these. These will deal with health and finance, as well as suitable accommodation, one or more absorbing hobbies, congenial friends and neighbours and finally an adequate philosophy of life. It is generally agreed that the most successful courses are small having between 12 and 20 students. This enables the tutor and lecturers to interact with the group and deal with their particular problems as well as dealing with the theoretical aspects of retirement. Course lecturers need careful briefing. The Pre-retirement Association has appropriate lecture notes available and these should be studied. It is important that lecturers concentrate on the positive aspects of retirement and on the gain and fulfilment that can be achieved during retirement. The negative and depressing aspects such as ill health and bereavement, poverty and loneliness must be faced in a positive manner, and ways of recognising and mitigating them suggested.

COMMUNITY SERVICES (Cases 1, 2, 6, 8 and 9)

The White Paper "Caring for People", on which the NHS and Community Care Act 1990 is based, states that elderly people should be enabled to "live as independently as possible in their own homes, or in 'homely' settings in the community". This policy is in accord with the wishes of the vast majority of the elderly, and places emphasis on the need for good community services to be available to the primary health care team. New legislation, in the Act also places a responsibility on the GP to examine all elderly over the age of 75 years, as well as taking steps to promote health positively (Chapter 1). There is no doubt that this will become a team effort with nurses and health visitors combining with the doctor to provide a service that aims at promoting health and preventing ill health and its consequences by early detection and the surveillance of high risk groups, such as the recently bereaved or recently discharged from hospital. The primary health care team of doctor, his surgery staff of practice manager, receptionists, and nurses are supported by the home nursing service, health visitors, community psychiatric nurses, community physiotherapists, continence advisory service and services provided by the LA social services department. These will include social workers, occupational therapists, and probably various liaison officers with varying responsibilities, such as liaison with district health authority (HA), residential and nursing homes in the private and voluntary sector, district housing authorities, agencies (private and voluntary) providing home care services such as home help, laundry, meals, sitting and visiting, close care, care and repair and the numerous other entrepreneurial schemes, such as Macmillan nurses or Age Concern "shoppers" (Case 9), which may operate in some districts. Other services such as day centres, luncheon clubs, equipment stores may also be provided by the LA itself or by voluntary agencies. In addition to all these the HA's geriatric and psychogeriatric services will provide community support in the form of domiciliary consultations, day hospital treatment, respite care in cases unsuitable for residential or nursing home, and some items of equipment.

VOLUNTARY SERVICES

Most voluntary organisations are charities registered with the Charity Commission which is responsible for monitoring their operation. As a result some charities are limited companies and as such subject to the Company Act, the charity's trustees being the company directors.

As such, the effectiveness and efficiency of many voluntary organisations has been improved considerably. Those voluntary organisations which concentrate on providing services to the elderly can play an important part in the overall spectrum of care. However, considerable mistrust of the volunteer still exists in the statutory sector. The reason for this is that volunteers may prove unreliable, not always providing the support or service that has been promised. This has changed somewhat in that many voluntary organisations have a central core of paid staff that direct the voluntary effort under the direction of an executive committee comprised of volunteers. The core funding for much of this central staff is provided by a grant from the LA who, therefore, have some control over the service(s) being provided. The disadvantage of this arrangement to the voluntary organisation is that the grant may only given on a yearly basis, so that forward planning is difficult. With the implementation of the NHS and Community Care Act in April 1993 this situation should improve. Then, the voluntary agency will be able to act as a "provider of services" competing for a contract with the LA to provide a defined service for a period of time, usually 3 years. This should enable the voluntary organisation to plan its services on a longer term basis, thereby improving efficiency. Some of the leading organisations working in the field of the care of the elderly are Age Concern (England), Age Concern (Scotland), Help the Aged, The Centre for Policy on Ageing, The Carers National Association, Distressed Gentlefolks Association, the Abbeyfield Society, the Salvation Army and many others. They provide services covering a very wide range from general support, such as housing with care or travelling day centres, to personal services, like advocacy and visiting and sitting schemes. The major role of the voluntary organisation is to seek out and meet unmet need until such a time as that service proves unnecessary or is provided by the state because it has proved to be indispensable and needed universally.

SPECIALIST HOUSING FOR THE ELDERLY

A proportion of the housing stock of all district housing authorities will be occupied by elderly people. In addition each housing authority provides some housing specially for the elderly. This falls into two categories, Category 1, which consists of housing which has been designed and built for the elderly, and Category 2, whereby flatlets and maisonettes are usually grouped together and the fabric supervised by a warden. Recently it has been recognized that provision of additional support, with the help of social services and the health services, enables the frail and dependent elderly to remain within this setting thereby saving a place in a residential home. This provides a more cost-effective service as well as one which is more appreciated by the individual. Such an arrangement has sometimes been called Category $2\frac{1}{2}$ housing or Part $2\frac{1}{2}$ accommodation. It is perhaps better called housing for the frail, dependent elderly or very sheltered housing. This type of housing provides 24 hour warden cover and the wardens, usually, have had some training in the care of the elderly and are in a position to alert and mobilise the necessary health or social services when needed. A recent review of very sheltered housing carried out by the Age Concern Institute of Social Gerontology suggests that very sheltered housing is an effective way in which the elderly can maintain their independence yet receive extra care. When this happens, it can be truly said that housing is the bricks and mortar of community care.

Similarly some voluntary organisations have established housing associations for this purpose. These then have applied to the Housing Corporation for a grant from their "special needs" housing allocation (currently about 15% of their annual government grant). Any application must be supported by the LA, with regard to the need for such specialist housing and accommodation. Some housing associations, such as the Anchor Housing Association, also provide some care in their complexes. There is no doubt that such specialist housing has enabled elderly people to remain in a "homely" setting in the community for much longer than might have been otherwise.

All such special category sheltered housing is linked to a warden by some form of *alarm system*. Modern communication systems provide an extension of the alarm system so that a link can be established between the elderly and their carers, via telephone or radio link. While such a link will undoubtedly provide psychological support for both carer and client, it is likely that these systems are overvalued. Their cost/effectiveness needs to be weighed against other simpler systems and methods of supervision.

RESIDENTIAL ACCOMMODATION (Cases 4, 5 and 8)

A small number of people cannot survive in the community, even in very sheltered accommodation, and require the hotel type of residential home that is provided by the LA social services department under Part 3 of the National Assistance Act 1947. The recommended provision was for 25 places per 1000 elderly over 65 years. Such homes cost a lot both to build and to run, and by 1977 many LAs were reviewing their policy in this respect. Revision of the supplementary benefits scheme in 1980 meant that a "reasonable" board and lodging allowance could be paid to old people in private residential homes. This resulted in an enormous expansion of the private sector, beginning in 1981. This in particular tended to affect those districts with high retirement populations and where the statutory provision of places was low. Hence the number of residents per 1000 population over 65 years in private residential homes in the south and south-west of England was approximately twice the national average of 7·5. The number of private home places had increased to over 160 000 by 1991, according to the 1992 Laing and Buisson *Care of the Elderly*: Market Survey. However, recent policy decisions have tended to move the care of the elderly away from this type of institution and this may be the cause for the drop in the rate of annual increase from 9% in 1990 to

4% in 1991. In spite of this, demand for residential care is expected to grow and it is anticipated that an additional 89 000 places will be needed between 1991 and 2000. This is due to the expected increase in the 85-year-old population, since it is estimated that at any one time 15 to 20% of this population are in some form of care.

LONG-TERM HOSPITAL CARE

An individual may develop such severe mental or physical handicap that his care places intolerable stress on those looking after him at home or in residential accommodation. When this happens he should be admitted to a specially designed unit that has nursing facilities together with remedial therapy and an activities organiser, so that individuals are encouraged to maximise their abilities. This particular category of care has been long neglected, for there is little more that can be done for these patients from the curative medical standpoint, even though they can live lives of considerable quality if they are given the chance by being adequately supported by health professionals and others. Since this unit will now become the patient's home, its aim should be to ensure the individual's autonomy placing the emphasis more on leisure activities than on traditional hospital care (Chapter 9). It is no easy task to organise, plan, run and maintain high standards in such a home. Fostering autonomy means involving the patients (residents) in the running of the home, difficult when many will have impaired intellectual function, but residents committees are possible and add to the interest of all, helping to normalise life. Also creative roles can be given to residents even when they are severely handicapped. If this can be achieved, the individual can retain his identity and self-respect and feel that he still has a useful part to play in life. A considerable social work role remains to be explored in this particular field.

Where this type of care should be best undertaken is debatable. Currently, many district health authorities have passed the responsibility for this type of care over to the private sector, but if the home is situated within the NHS a conscious effort has to be made by all staff to remember that the "patients" are *residents*. While there is no doubt that the ambience provided by a modern nursing home is infinitely superior to the geriatric ward in the old poor law hospital, it is doubtful if the care is better. The most important aspect of the care of these patients is the attitude of those who are doing the caring. In addition to providing activities and fostering autonomy, special attention must be paid to the living environment and the food. The former needs to provide a homely setting with privacy as well as space, light and warmth. With the latter particular attention must be paid to meals. Research has shown that these residents are frequently undernourished. This may be for many reasons; e.g. they have not been given enough to eat: they have not been given long enough to eat the food provided: food is unpalatable and unattractive: the food is cold when it should be hot: all courses are served at the same time. A good chef, catering officer and dietitian who communicate with each other are essential and meals need to be planned and prescribed with the same care as medicines as part of the care plan. The skill needed to provide good long-term care is special and may not necessarily be that of the doctor. But, it must be remembered that long-term continuing care is not a cheap option. High quality care costs £350–450/week depending on the part of the country.

A perennial problem of long-term care is whether people with mental impairment should be mixed with those who are physically incapacitated but mentally normal. One of the stigmas of the long-stay hospital is that the patients are all "geriatric", an adjective which frequently has pejorative connotations. There is no doubt that many patients in long-stay units have brain damage and therefore impaired intellectual performance; this is usually coupled with physical incapacity so that the patient is immobile. Under these circumstances a patient is normally accepted in a medical long-stay unit where about three-quarters of the patients will be the same. If, however, the patient is mobile and therefore liable to wander or has other unacceptable behaviour he should be cared for in a psychiatric long-stay unit. In either case the unit should be so organised to help the individual achieve his maximum potential. Where such division of patients into separate units is not possible, arrangements should be made to care for the different categories in separate clinical areas.

FURTHER READING

Audit Commission (1992). *Community Care: Managing the Cascade of Change.* London: HMSO.

Bromley, D.B. (ed.) (1984). *Gerontology—Social and Behavioural Perspectives.* London: Croom Helm.

Marshall, M. (1985). *Social Work with Old People*. London: Macmillan Education.

McClymont, M. and Thomas, S. (1986). *Health Visiting and the Elderly*. Edinburgh: Churchill Livingstone.

Parker, R.A. (1987). *The Elderly and Residential Care. Australian Lessons for Britain*. Aldershot: Gower.

Redfern, S.J. (1991). *Nursing Elderly People*. Edinburgh: Churchill Livingstone.

Royal College of Physicians and British Geriatrics Society (1992). *High Quality Long-term Care for Elderly People*. London: Royal College of Physicians.

Wells, N. and Freer, C. (ed.) (1988). *The Ageing Population. Burden or Challenge*. London: Macmillan.

Your Rights. Published annually by Age Concern (England).

CHAPTER 5   Treatment and management of the elderly patient

INTRODUCTION

The first four chapters of this book have stressed the importance of accurate assessment of the elderly patient. This not only means clinical investigation and diagnosis but also the physical, mental and social assessment of the individual's capacity which is essential in the effective planning of treatment and management.

Elderly patients referred to the hospital geriatric service may be seen and treated as outpatients, day-patients or inpatients. Out-patients are usually referred by a GP for an opinion on a clinical or clinico-social condition. The patient will usually be seen at the outpatient department by the consultant who will collate the infor-mation given him by the GP, the patient and, given the patient's permission, any relative or friend who may have accompanied them. He may then be able to suggest a solution to the problem raised by the GP. However to do this may require the performance of various investigations on the patient as an outpatient or, if this is not practicable, as a day-patient or inpatient; many hospitals now have 5-day wards which can be used to admit patients for a whole series of "programmed" investigations. Recently discharged patients may also be followed up for a limited time, as outpatients, in order to monitor progress and ensure that therapeutic goals already set are being achieved and maintained. This task, however, should be handed over to the GP as soon as possible.

For each of the case histories (pp. 1–35) a problem list has been constructed to show some of the possible effects that could result from the medical problems. Various actions which can be taken to counteract these effects are given in the third column of the prob-lem list. These lists are not intended to be comprehensive and the discerning, imaginative reader will be able to add to the number of possible effects and, therefore, the possible actions it may be necessary to take. As can be seen from these case histories many professionals, belonging to different specialties and with differing skills, are involved in the treatment of the patient. While many patients respond well to the treatment prescribed, some present complex problems of management. Since the professionals may need to collaborate with each other, the management of the treatment will need careful planning and considerable cross-consultation will have to take place. The objective in all cases is to try and achieve optimum performance with the greatest degree of comfort. Therefore, the patient, his relatives and those who will continue to look after him ouside of the hospital will need to be consulted. Communication can therefore be difficult, and it is important that the management of all cases is as efficient as possible and that time is not wasted because one or more members of the therapeutic team are not sure of their exact role.

Since the elderly are often frail and severely disabled, it is most important to set goals which are attainable. Expecting too much may engender a sense of failure which may negate further treatment, particularly remedial therapy aimed at rehabilitation and re-enablement. The goals must be clearly defined and understood by all members of the therapeutic team, and the patient and his relatives, so that the response of the elderly patient to treatment can be monitored accurately and appropriate adjustments made at regular intervals.

THE CASE CONFERENCE (Cases 1 and 8)

For the inpatient or day-patient a case conference may be essential if efficient treatment and management plans are to be made (Figure 5.1). With so many people involved in the treatment and management of a single patient chaos could arise unless their actions are carefully coordinated and understood. Hence, the need for a case conference where details can be discussed and the varying assessments and views of the health care professionals stated and discussed. The doctor as the leader can then agree with the various members of the team the role that each will play in relation to the patient, decide the priorities and set the therapeutic goals. These, for the sake of clarity, should be described in simple "performance" terms, e.g. standing unsupported, walking with a stick, etc. As can be seen from the problem lists, elderly patients have many problems, some of which they recognise and many they do not. Problems which may seem of prime importance to the therapeutic team may be relatively unimportant to the patient, whereas a relatively simple overlooked problem, such as a corn or a deformed toenail (onychogryphosis) or the inability to perform some specific task, may cause the greatest hardship not only to the patient but also to the carer. For instance an 82-year-old lady with a left hemiparesis due to an old stroke became bedfast, incontinent and developed a small pressure sore because her inability to walk was attributed to her stroke, rather than her painful deformed toenails which the chiropodist had no difficulty in treating. In deciding priorities for treatment, the wishes and views of patients must be sought since the major objective of all treatment is to improve the quality of their life and this can only be achieved by a partnership of the patient and therapeutic team. The more rapidly this can be done the better it is for the individual. A checklist similar to that shown in Table 5.1 will help to ensure that information is complete.

It is beyond the scope of this handbook to discuss the rights of patients and the ethical problems that may arise during treatment. But, it must be stressed that the rights of individuals must always be remembered and their wishes respected. The elderly frequently have great difficulty in making up their minds and often the more information that they are given the more difficult it becomes. Explanations must be simple and plenty of time allowed to discuss the pros and cons. Relatives may be invaluable in helping the team

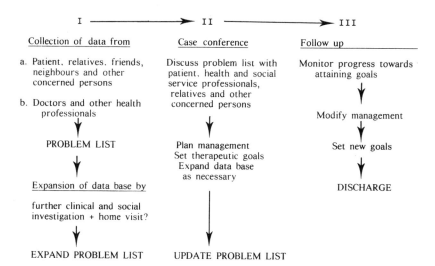

Figure 5.1   Flow diagram to illustrate the place of the case conference

Table 5.1   Case conference checklist

Medical problems: diagnosis and treatment
Social state and interaction with medical state
Special problems: hearing
                 speech
                 vision
Mental state: confused
             depressed
             alert
Urinary control
Bowel function
Teeth
Feet
Physical capacity: feeding   dressing
                  sitting in bed/chair   toileting
                  transferring bed/chair   bathing
                  standing   household tasks
                  walking: with help   cooking ability
                          with aid   shopping
                          alone
Set goals for attainment
Information to be discussed with patient and ?relatives

to ensure that the patient has understood what is happening, but it is most important that the patient's permission is given before anything is discussed with relatives. While most old people are only too pleased for their relatives to be involved, there are some who will refuse on the grounds that it is none of their business. Patient confidentiality and autonomy is as important in this age group as in any other adult group (Cases 5 and 9).

The case conference, although time consuming, is essential if the best overall results are to be achieved for it provides a good forum in which to discuss ethical problems and propound varying views concerning correct patient care. As such, it is a most useful teaching and training ground for medical, nursing, therapy and social work students as well as providing a base for the continuing audit of progress. It also provides a continuous record of the management of a variety of clinical and clinico-social problems which can be invaluable when auditing process and outcomes.

DRUG THERAPY

While drugs play a very important part in the management of many medical problems, drug therapy itself is not without its drawbacks in the elderly. In recent years a considerable amount of work has been done on the effect ageing has on the way in which drugs are absorbed, distributed, metabolised and excreted (pharmacokinetics) and on the effect drugs have on target organs (pharmacodynamics). When one considers the alterations which occur in various physiological systems with ageing it is hardly surprising that drugs may have different effects on older people than they do on the young, and may be absorbed, metabolised and excreted in different ways and at different rates. The following sections deal with some of these physiological changes in more detail.

Pharmacokinetics of Drugs

In prescribing drugs for elderly patients it is important to bear in mind some of the changes which occur in their absorption, metabolism and excretion. Adverse drug reactions are very common in old people and can occur either as a result of the patient being given too large a dose or by altered pharmacokinetic handling resulting in higher drug levels and a prolonged drug life. It should be emphasised that some of these changes are of academic interest rather than practical importance. The effects of ageing on pharmacokinetics should be put in the context of the major effects which multiple pathology and drug interactions may have on this process. Finally if an elderly patient on drug treatment develops new symptoms, the doctor's first thought must be "could a drug be causing this?"

Absorption

Ageing has very little effect on drug absorption. Indeed changes in liver function mean that less of the drug is removed as it passes from the portal system through the liver (first pass metabolism). This means that many drugs, achieve higher initial plasma levels. Moreover, gastrointestinal motility may be altered, as a result of ageing changes in the gut, or due to the effect of other drugs (e.g. anticholinergics, laxatives) so that drug absorption may be affected and peak levels may take longer to achieve. For example, this might be important in the use of a hypnotic, where delayed absorption may prolong the period of sleeplessness, and have a sedative effect the following day.

Metabolism

Age-related changes in enzymes involved in oxidative metabolism mean that it takes longer for the body to eliminate drugs mainly metabolised by this route. There is less of a problem with agents eliminated by conjugation in the liver, since this process does not change with age. There is conflicting evidence on the effects of ageing on drug acetylation. Indeed genetic differences have far more of an effect on this process than ageing.

Volume of Distribution

Concentration of drugs in old people may be affected by a reduction in muscle mass and an increase in the proportion of fat mass. The apparent volume of distribution of mainly water soluble drugs is reduced in the elderly in proportion to the reduction in lean body mass; the result is to enhance the drug's "concentration". Conversely, a fat soluble drug dissolved within an increased volume of adipose tissue will have a lower concentration.

Protein Binding

A low serum albumin concentration means that less protein is available for binding a drug so that the proportion of the free and, consequently, active drug is increased. Ageing itself causes only a marginal fall in the serum albumin concentration, but the process is often exacerbated by disease. A reduction of binding sites on the albumin molecule may also occur with age, thereby also increasing free (active) drug levels. Different drugs may compete for available protein binding sites thus enhancing the activity of one or both drugs.

Elimination

Diminished renal excretion undoubtedly plays a large part in the retention of some drugs (Chapter 13). The formulation of most drugs as weak bases may also be a factor in their defective elimination. It is well known that basic drugs are better reabsorbed by the kidney if the urine is alkaline. Many elderly subjects live on reduced incomes and have low protein intakes, so that their urine tends to be alkaline. Further, old people often drink less fluid and consequently pass less urine. Both these factors will lead to higher blood drug concentrations.

Basic Principles

1. All drugs should be considered potentially harmful to the elderly patient. Drugs are given to relieve symptoms and, consequently, before a drug is prescribed, the symptom must be viewed in relation to the distress it is causing, and the adverse effects of the drug to be used weighed against the distress caused by the symptom.

Ankle swelling is a good example, as it is a relatively common occurrence in old age and has many causes. Diuretics are commonly prescribed to relieve the system, often without reference to the cause, and adverse reactions that may occur, such as urinary incontinence, a fall in blood pressure after standing or taking exercise (Chapter 10, "Postural hypotension"), a reduction in glucose tolerance unmasking or exacerbating diabetes mellitus, or potassium depletion with associated weakness and lethargy. If the ankle swelling is related to heart failure then almost certainly the diuretic was correctly prescribed. Ankle swelling is often due to immobility, and is then treated better by encouraging exercise, elevating the legs whenever possible, and/or using graded pressure stockings and/or bandages. In these patients a diuretic has only a limited effect so that its benefits do not justify the risk of side effects.

Having decided that a drug is necessary it is essential to monitor the effect of that drug to ensure that it is not causing any ill effects and has indeed achieved the initial therapeutic objective—if not it should be reviewed, stopped or changed. Figure 5.2 provides a flow chart which applies the above principles to the management of individual patients. The patient's compliance should also be confirmed. It is important to remember that higher blood concentrations per dose may result from altered metabolism and diminished excretion so that a lower or less frequent dose of the drug may be needed.

2. When giving a drug treat the patient as an individual and titrate the dose of the drug in relation to the patient's response and the predetermined objectives. The use of L-dopa in the treatment of Parkinson's disease (Chapter 8) is a good example of this principle. The elderly patient will often suffer adverse effects from L-dopa if the dose given is too large or the increment made too quickly, and initial doses may be so small that in younger patients they would seem homeopathic. Sometimes, when there is a narrow window between effectiveness and toxicity, it may be helpful to measure blood levels.

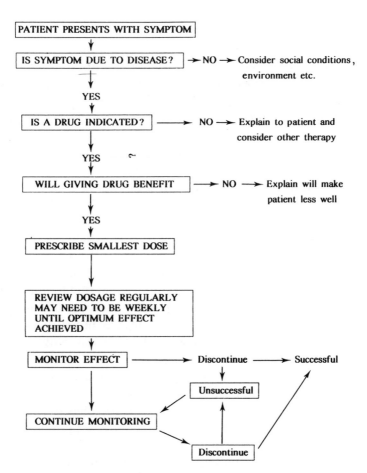

Figure 5.2   Flow chart to show steps in prescription

Examples of drugs in which this can be important include digoxin, theophylline and gentamicin.

3. Large loading doses are rarely necessary unless a rapid response is needed.   For instance, the normal loading doses of digoxin needed in the younger patient will be as effective in the older patient. However, the dose necessary to maintain therapeutic response may be as low as 125 μg and rarely exceeds 250 μg daily, the response to a particular dose being dependent upon both body build and renal function.

4. Drug regimens must be kept constantly under review.   Since old people suffer from multiple pathology it frequently may be necessary to use more than one drug in a patient, and the possibility of interaction between one drug and another must always be borne in mind. Moreover the elderly often self-prescribe and self-medicate. Community studies have shown that many elderly people, designated as "healthy" by their GPs, are taking three or four different pharmacological preparations, some of which are unknown to their GP. The use of "over the counter" preparations by old people is often entirely justifiable. Indeed the workload of general practitioners would be increased substantially if patients did not resort to these for minor ailments. Their use, however, must be remembered and identified when doctors prescribe drugs for the elderly patient.

5. Repeat prescriptions given to elderly patients should be reviewed every 3 months.   While there are many elderly patients who require drugs for life in order to keep their medical condition under control, e.g. diabetes, asthma etc., their prescription should be reviewed regularly. It should be recognised also that some conditions do get better, for example it has been shown that in many patients diuretics can be discontinued without ill effects, as can antidepressants. Prescriptions should be continued only if they are genuinely thought to be essential. A trial of drug withdrawal is often helpful, especially before deciding to add further drugs to a complex regimen.

6. Keep drug regimens simple.   Elderly patients may have difficulty in managing complex drug regimens. Only three or four preparations can be given successfully at any one time to the majority of patients. Complex regimens also increase the incidence of drug side effects and interactions. It is unwise to prescribe more than this number of drugs if self-administration is to be relied upon. Fortunately for the elderly, omission of medication is the most frequent error. If this were not so the incidence of symptoms due to the ill effect of drugs (iatrogenic disease) would be considerably higher. If compliance is very important and self-medication has to be relied upon, once or twice daily regimens are likely to be the most effective. Nevertheless, there is debate as to whether drugs taken less frequently do improve compliance, for some feel that if a patient forgets a dose in a once daily regimen he will be more likely to run into trouble than if he misses one out of four doses. In many cases it may be necessary to positively choose not to treat a condition or symptom which has a low priority assigned to it by either the doctor or the patient, or preferably, both.

REHABILITATION AND THE ADJUSTMENT OF THE ENVIRONMENT   (Cases 1, 2, 3, and 8)

While drugs can be used to control the individual's internal environment his ability to perform ordinary acts of daily living are probably of even greater importance to him, and while doctors and nurses have an important part to play in the adjustment of an individual's internal environment, the whole team, but especially the remedial therapists, have an important role in adjusting his external one. By active educative exercises, the physiotherapist can increase muscle strength, as well as the range of joint and limb movement, thereby improving movements which will enable the individual to increase his functional abilities. The main objective is to restore his independence and enable him to perform the essential acts of daily life. In simple terms this means getting up out of bed, getting dressed, walking to the lavatory, using it, walking back to bed, getting undressed, and getting back into bed. The physiotherapist will bear this in mind when treating the patient and set appropriate goals, so that the patient will achieve independence in due course. As previously mentioned, goals set must be achievable so that the patient's morale is boosted by treatment and he is encouraged to progress to the next phase. Mobility may be increased by the prescription of various walking aids, while patients who are unable to walk may be capable of being taught to lead independent lives in a wheelchair. Also the individual may be limited in his ability to overcome obstacles, such as steps and stairs, which may exist at home. In these cases the therapist must visit the home to make a first-hand assessment in order to find a solution to that problem which interferes with the patient's ability to live independently at home and thereby hinders his discharge.

Similarly, the occupational therapist has an essential role to play in training him to overcome the difficulties he may encounter in daily life, prescribing and teaching him to use any aids that are necessary. She/he must collaborate closely with the physiotherapist in order to restore the patient's independence and achieve his discharge from hospital. Such skills as cooking, housekeeping and shopping are luxuries which, however desirable, should not prevent discharge, since home support in the form of meals-on-wheels, home help and the laundry service can be provided through the social services department. Nevertheless, it has to be accepted that frail, disabled elderly people who have recently been in hospital are likely to have many accidents at home. Falls can occur as a result of unsteadiness and some simple precautions should be taken to mitigate these if they do occur. Patients should be actively taught how to pick themselves up off the floor. If this cannot be achieved, appropriate alarm systems should be devised and blankets kept within reach of the floor so that patients can keep warm if they have to remain on the floor overnight or until help arrives.

The amount of time a physiotherapist or occupational therapist can spend with an individual patient is limited, and it is thus essential that, while the patient is in hospital, the nurse should take an active part in the rehabilitation process. Examples include encouraging the patient to dress rather than be dressed; getting him to go to the lavatory rather than use a commode; and ensuring that he spends as much time as possible practising walking. In the geriatric setting, the nurse in addition to fulfilling the traditional roles must also be a "nurse therapist" and a full member of the rehabilitation team thereby reinforcing the work done by other professionals (Chapter 8).

ANAESTHESIA AND SURGERY

Many doctors other than the geriatrician are likely to be involved in the care of the elderly patient. It has been estimated that about half of those people at present aged 65 years will require surgery at some time during their remaining lifetime. Surgery, and therefore, anaesthesia is important and will become even more so in the future. This applies more in some surgical specialties, such as urology, orthopaedics and ophthalmology, in which about half the admissions are over 65 years.

It is not possible in a short handbook to cover all the problems that may arise in the management of the surgical patient. The reader must refer to appropriate texts. Careful assessment of the patient as outlined in this and the preceding chapters together with some knowledge of the ageing process is essential if management is going to be successful and the patient discharged home as soon as possible. It is important to remember that while age is almost never a bar to surgery, the elderly patient wants to spend as short a time in hospital as possible. The modern anaesthetist is so skilled that there is hardly an elderly patient who cannot have an anaesthetic. Nevertheless postoperative complications are more likely to occur in older subjects and in those who have preoperative medical problems. Hence, while nearly 60% of those aged 65–74 years will have no postoperative complication, only about 30% of those aged over 75 years will have none. Similarly, while 60% of those with no preoperative medical problem will have no complications, less than 30% of those with three or more preoperative medical problems will have none. As has already been stated (Chapter 3) multiple pathology is common in old age. Cardiac and respiratory complications are the most common postoperative occurrences and are more likely to occur in patients who have a history of disease in these systems, regardless of their age. The amount of special investigation needed before surgery is undertaken will depend on the severity of the cardiac or respiratory problem. The importance of careful assessment in these subjects cannot be overemphasised. Similarly, renal function and control of homeostasis (Chapter 13) are important in the postoperative period, while assessment of nutritional state should be undertaken and corrected, if necessary, preoperatively.

Close cooperation between the surgical/anaesthetic team and the geriatric medical team should be encouraged. Such collaboration will promote research and knowledge. Early mobilisation with adequate pain relief and specialist measures to prevent bed sores can do much to speed recovery and shorten the hospital stay. The organisation of joint clinical areas between either orthopaedic or urological surgeons and geriatricians, in some districts, has been shown to be an effective way of improving patient management.

BED SORES

A bed sore occurs when prolonged pressure cuts off the blood supply to an area of skin and subcutaneous tissue. For example, a pressure of 60 mmHg lasting for 60 minutes is sufficient to produce a pressure sore. On admission of the patient, the skin should be examined carefully for evidence of reddening, excoriation, discoloration or ulceration at those parts of the body where pressure sores (decubitus ulcers) are most likely to occur (pressure points). These are shown in Table 5.2. The incidence of pressure sores is directly related to immobility. Studies of the sleeping patient have shown that sores are unlikely to occur if the patient has 20 spontaneous movements or more during a 7 hour period. People tend to move spontaneously when they become uncomfortable, and the discomfort produced by pressure on a pressure point will bring about this automatic movement. Conditions which immobilise the patient, render the skin insensitive or diminish its natural resistance predispose to the development of a sore. Reduced movement is particularly likely to occur in patients with a poor general condition, and in those who are subnourished, oversedated or comatose, incontinent, or who suffer a chronic neurological illness.

Pressure sores are unpleasant and painful, difficult to heal, and may keep the patient in hospital for a long time. The cost of treating sores has been estimated as £450 million/year (1992) and the incidence may be as high as 35% in some vulnerable groups. Prevention is possible and can be achieved by identifying those at risk and instituting appropriate measures. These include the following:

Table 5.2   Common pressure sore sites

Trochanter
Ischial tuberosity
Ischial crest
Sacrum
Spinous process
Scapula
Heel
Malleoli
Elbow

1. Changing the patient's position at least every 2 hours, so that pressure over the "pressure points" is never allowed to reach a level which will cause a sore to develop.
2. Making sure the skin, at potential pressure sites, is dry and clean; the use of a zinc based cream may help to act as a "barrier" to moisture and infection.
3. Giving attention to the patient's position in bed or chair so that the risk of "shearing" a blood vessel connecting deep and subcutaneous tissue is kept to a minimum. "Shearing" is more likely to occur if the patient is nursed in the semi-recumbent position.
4. Ensuring the general condition of the patient is as good as possible by correcting anaemia, avoiding dehydration, promoting good nutrition, and encouraging movement and exercise at the earliest possible moment.
5. Avoiding conditions likely to produce pressure sores, e.g. "long lies" on stretchers in ambulances or casualty department, or other hard surfaces such as X-ray tables and operating tables.
6. Using nursing aids such as special cushions and mattresses, such as the intermittent pressure mattress, or even a special "flotation" bed which will keep pressure to a minimum. Sheep skins may also be helpful in that they may prevent sweating and keep the skin dry and cool. These aids are not a substitute for early mobilisation and encouraging movement.

Once a pressure sore has developed the treatments are legion. Almost every practitioner has his own regime. The important principles are to control sepsis and remove dead tissue (eschar) by cutting it away until bleeding occurs or the patient complains of pain. Once this is done the sore will heal by epithelialisation. In the case of large sores, reconstructive plastic surgery may be possible, once the sore is clean. A plastic surgeon's opinion should be sought if sores are slow to heal, for surgery may speed healing, so that the patient is discharged more quickly.

FURTHER READING

Andrews, K. (1991). *Rehabilitation of the Older Adult*. London: Edward Arnold.
Border, D.L. (1990). *Pressure Sores*. London: Macmillan.

Cartwright, A. and Smith, C. (1988). *Elderly People, Their Drugs and Their Doctors*. London: Routledge & Kegan Paul.

Crosby, D.L., Rees, G.A.D. and Seymour, D.G. (ed) (1992). *The Ageing Surgicial Patient*. Chichester: Wiley.

Davies, P.M. (1990). *Right in the Middle*. Berlin: Springer Verlag.

Denham, M.J. (1991). *Care of the Long Stay Elderly Patient*, 2nd edn. London: Croom Helm.

Denham, M.J. and George, C.F. (1990). Drugs in old age. British Medical Bulletin **46**: 1–299.

Mulley, G. (1991). *Everyday Aids and Appliances*. London: British Medical Journal.

Mulley, G. (1992). *More Everyday Aids and Appliances*. London: British Medical Journal.

Seymour, G. (1986). *Medical Assessment of the Surgical Patient*. London: Croom Helm.

CHAPTER 6   It's just old age

Although ageing is associated with some decline in organ and tissue function, most of the symptoms and disabilities afflicting old people result from disease. Most laymen and many professionals, however, consider that failing faculties, severe disability and multiple aches and pains are inevitable and irreversible accompaniments of ageing. A 40-year-old man who experiences sudden onset of chest pain requests an urgent home visit from his doctor. If an 85-year-old woman experiences the same symptom she is likely to shrug her shoulders and say "What can you expect? It's just old age." It is vital that the general public and professionals should be educated in the differences between the effects of ageing and those of disease. Failure to appreciate these can have disastrous consequences both for individuals and for the heavily stretched supporting services.

HEARING (Case 2)

Loss of hearing (presbyacusis) is a common but not inevitable accompaniment of ageing. It is partly due to the natural loss of irreplaceable receptors in the cochlea, atrophy of the organ of Corti and other structural changes. Environment may also be of major importance. At the one extreme is the country dweller who has lived in a quiet, relatively noise free environment and who has retained excellent hearing; conversely, there is the worker in heavy industry who may become deaf in late middle age. Surveys show that about 30% of old people over the age of 65 years have some loss of hearing.

Although their hearing is impaired for all frequencies of sound, old people have most difficulty in picking up high-pitched sounds. This means that, even if a hearing aid is used, sounds may be badly distorted.

In the cochlea the receptors for soft sounds are more severely degenerated than those for loud ones, which may account for a normal voice being inaudible, but shouting being painful—a phenomenon known as "recruitment". The reasonable request, "Please speak up, I am hard of hearing", may be followed by the irate complaint, "There's no need to shout. I am not deaf." Slow, well articulated speech with the speaker's facial movements clearly visible to the patient is the answer to this problem.

The patient also may have difficulty in focusing onto sounds. This manifests itself at social gatherings where difficulty may arise in separating the conversation of a neighbour from the background noise. It may also account for the state of confusion which the hoot of a horn induces in an elderly person crossing the road.

The frequency of presbyacusis should not lead to the neglect of other possible causes of deafness in old age. Old people were brought up in a pre-antibiotic era when middle ear infections were extremely common. At a more mundane level many elderly suffer from deafness, dizziness and buzzing in their ears simply because their external auditory canals are full of wax.

The diagnosis of presbyacusis is made from the configuration of the pure tone audiogram, and in many cases, the loss of hearing may be greater in one ear. Speech frequency varies between 500 and 2000 hertz (Hz) and hearing loss is greatest in the higher frequencies, so that the sibilant sounds tend to be lost. When the hearing loss exceeds 35 decibels (dB) a hearing aid should be prescribed. This often improves communication but many old people are reluctant to use such an instrument. They may be diffident about admitting they are deaf, or have difficulty in learning the rather complex technique involved in using the instrument. Batteries may go flat. Hideous whines may occur when inadequate fitting of the earpiece allows sounds to be transmitted back from the earpiece to the receiver, and there may be difficulty in adjusting the instrument to pick up conversation while keeping background noise to a minimum.

It is unfortunate that although there have been great technical developments and a major expansion in the provision of hearing aids, much less attention has been given to training patients in their use. Careful instruction on the use of the aid is essential, and regular follow-up is important if effective use of the aid is to be achieved. In the absence of such formal education, doctors, nurses and relatives must take on the task of helping and encouraging old people to use their aids. Many old people can learn to lip read and should be taught this whenever possible, but unfortunately lip reading is another subject which has been neglected in planning services for the elderly deaf and few formal teaching classes are held. This neglect has been partly due to the attitude held by providers of services that the elderly are unable to learn new tasks, in other words ageist attitudes. This is a pity, since deafness is perhaps the worst disability one can suffer, for one can be deprived of contact with other people's minds. This increases loneliness and can lead to psychiatric disorders.

A major advance in supporting deaf elderly patients has been the development of professional hearing therapists (Case 2). They have a valuable part to play in the care of the elderly deaf. They can act as counsellors and teachers to patients as well as training others, including volunteers, to perform these functions: visiting people in their own homes, allaying their fears and teaching them to get the maximum benefit from their aids, as well as teaching their relatives about the problems that face the deaf. Though the profession has been in existence for over a decade, many health authorities have yet to appoint a hearing therapist. This is a pity since the service they provide is very cost effective, particularly when it is community orientated, and run by the volunteers they have recruited and trained.

VISION

Presbyopia

Ageing is invariably accompanied by deteriorating vision, in which changes in the elasticity and translucency of the lens play an important part. Reduced elasticity interferes with accommodation so that, though distance vision remains intact, close vision becomes blurred. The change develops quite rapidly in early middle age, but can be corrected by fitting convex lenses.

Cataract

Lens opacities tend to develop with age. A variety of patterns may be produced (Figure 6.1). The process is a consequence of ageing but it may be accelerated in some conditions (e.g. diabetes mellitus), in which cataracts may occur in middle rather than old age.

Lens extraction is the only effective treatment. In the past considerable problems were encountered in balancing vision between treated and untreated eyes. This problem has been resolved by inserting an artificial lens at the time of extraction. The modern operation consists of extracting the lens leaving the posterior capsule intact, cleaning it and inserting an acrylic artificial lens into the empty capsule. This procedure gives excellent visual results and has a very low incidence of complications. Also it has the advantage of being able to be done, using a local anaesthetic, in a cooperative patient, as a day surgery case, thereby avoiding admission to hospital.

Impaired Dark Adaptation

Retinal changes make it difficult for old eyes to adapt from bright to dark surroundings, which creates problems for old people who go out walking or driving at night, or where houses are inadequately illuminated by natural or artificial light. The problem is compounded by the fact that many old people have a defective sense of balance. Domestic hazards from this can be minimised by ensuring that there is adequate artificial and natural lighting, particularly on stairs and landings. Unseen hazards, such as loose bannisters, worn steps, trailing flexes, torn vinyl floor coverings, loose rugs or children's toys, must be avoided or corrected.

Glaucoma

Chronic simple (open angle) glaucoma is a disease characterised by an increase in the pressure of fluid within the eyeball. Although

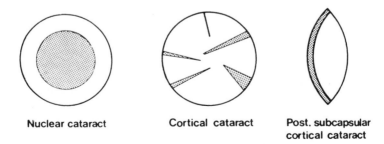

Nuclear cataract   Cortical cataract   Post. subcapsular
                                                     cortical cataract

Figure 6.1   Types of cataract occurring in old age

an increase in the intraocular pressure is not a concomitant of normal ageing, there is an increase in the prevalence of simple glaucoma with ageing. Table 6.1 summarises the features of the disease. Since the condition develops slowly, the patient often does not notice a gradual loss of peripheral vision; he may only notice that something is wrong when the macular damage prevents him from focusing on objects, by which time the visual change may have become irreversible.

Ideally, glaucoma should be identified as early as possible. Visual impairment should never be attributed to old age. All people involved in the care of the elderly should make sure that any deterioration in eyesight is reported and adequately investigated. Delay may be catastrophic.

Closed angle glaucoma usually presents as an acutely painful eye. There may have been a number of mild, self-limiting preceding attacks. The emergency treatment of closed angle glaucoma requires urgent 2% pilocarpine eye drops. The other eye is treated with 0.5% pilocarpine and the patient transferred to the ophthalmologist as soon as possible for iridectomy or specific drainage procedure.

Glaucoma is polygenic with no simple pattern of inheritance but is commoner in individuals for whom there is a family history of the condition. Screening those members of such families who are over 70 years may be justified. Screening for glaucoma in the elderly population in general is not justified. This is because there is no clear tonometric pressure which is predictive of glaucoma. If the level is set low the specificity is low, if high the sensitivity is low. Testing would merely place an extra load on overworked ophthalmic services.

The investigation and treatment of chronic glaucoma is a task for the ophthalmic surgeon. Diagnosis is made by a combination

Table 6.1   Features of chronic simple glaucoma (open angle glaucoma)

History	Perimetry
Insidious onset	Peripheral field defects
Tunnel vision	Macula not affected until late
No ocular discomfort	
Possible family history	
	Ophthalmoscopy
Tonometry	Cupping of optic disc
Increased intraocular pressure	Optic nerve atrophy

of tonometry, ophthalmoscopy and perimetry. Careful observation of the optic disc, particularly the size of the cup in relation to the disc, is most important in making an early diagnosis. First line treatment is aimed at reducing intraocular pressure, a topical beta-blocker, such as timolol, being prescribed. A miotic, such as pilocarpine, can be added to this if necessary. Alternatively adrenaline may be used in elderly asthmatics who may be intolerant of beta-blockers (Chapter 11). Other doctors should help by not prescribing drugs likely to aggravate the condition, particularly in those individuals who have a family history. In general, any agent which dilates the pupil is likely to increase intraocular pressures and many of the drugs used in the elderly have this side effect; they include tranquillisers, bladder relaxants and antidepressants. Clear communication between GP, ophthalmologist, geriatrician, nurse, patient and relatives is essential for good management.

Macular Degeneration (Case 2)

Old people may complain that while they are aware of their general surroundings they have great difficulty in seeing objects clearly. In other words, while they can find their way round the house, reading or watching television is impossible. These symptoms are often due to destruction of the macula, part of the retina responsible for focusing onto fine detail. The condition is due to disease of the local retinal blood vessels. If identified at a presymptomatic stage the condition can be arrested by laser photocoagulation of the offending blood vessels, but, once vision has become impaired, treatment is unlikely to be effective. Patients rarely present to the ophthalmologist at a presymptomatic stage, but close follow-up of patients with unilateral damage should ensure the early detection and treatment of the disease on the remaining healthy side. Patients will have to be warned to report any deterioration in vision to their doctor immediately. Photocoagulation, if needed, must be done urgently within a short time of the symptom occurring if it is to be successful in preventing deterioration. A delay of 2 weeks may mean that vision will be permanently affected. Some patients with more advanced disease benefit from strong reading glasses or using a magnifying glass.

Diabetic Retinopathy

Within 5 years of the diagnosis of non-insulin dependent diabetes mellitus (Chapter 13), one-third of the patients over the age of 65 years will have developed a retinopathy. This is characterised by hard circular exudates. Macular oedema is a particularly sinister complication in that it leads to central blindness. It is easily missed by standard ophthalmoscopy, and binocular stereoscopic equipment may be necessary for its diagnosis. An early sign of macular degeneration is a loss of central visual acuity. Proliferative neovascularisation is less common than in insulin dependent diabetes mellitus in younger age groups.

The risk of retinopathy can be reduced by tight control of blood glucose concentrations, and its progression arrested by laser photocoagulation.

Vascular Disease

This is a common cause of visual loss. Any part of the eye's circulation may be affected, retinal, choroidal or the most posterior part. The loss may be transient, often due to the passage of a platelet embolus (amaurosis fugax), or permanent. Occlusion of the arterial system causes a denser loss of vision than the venous system but is less common. Underlying conditions such as diabetes mellitus, hypertension, cranial arteritis (Chapter 7), glaucoma and migraine may be responsible and require treatment.

Retinal Detachment

Some retinal holes occur more frequently with age. There are two varieties, round holes, which are asymptomatic and are often a chance finding during ophthalmoscopy, and may not require any treatment, and the arrowhead tear usually occurring in the upper temporal quadrant. This is due to contraction of the vitreous which is attached to the apex of the tear. Shrinkage of the vitreous is a normal phenomenon of ageing. Vitreous opacities are common and are usually described as "floaters". They may be associated with crescentic flashes in the periphery of the field, which are often seen in conditions of low illumination and associated with head movements. The flashes are due to the detached vitreous hitting against the retina. The symptom is usually harmless, except where there is an abnormal attachment of the vitreous to the retina, in which case detachment may occur. In these cases chorioretinal adhesions may be created by the application of a cryoprobe or by laser photocoagulation. The flashes usually disappear after a time but the "floaters" persist, though they become less noticeable.

MOBILITY (Cases 1, 3, 4, 5, 6, 7, 8 and 10)

Many old people complain of decreasing mobility with increasing age. In the cases listed above, the reasons were—a pressure sore of the heel, Parkinson's disease (three cases), right hemiplegia, senile dementia, carer induced dependency, osteoarthritis of the spine and osteoarthritis of the knee. In these cases the loss of mobility was due to disease or a combination of diseases. However, ageing may also contribute, for progressive death of nerve cells controlling skeletal muscle occurs, and when these cells die they are not replaced. Examination may reveal muscle wasting and weakness with a resultant minor decline in function. There often is accelerated muscle wasting immediately after retirement. This is related to a reduction in physical exercise rather than neuronal loss. Health education can do a lot to prevent such deterioration. The form of exercise is less important than the fact that it is enjoyable. A few individuals may take up jogging, but many more prefer to take up golf, go hillwalking or take the dog for a walk (see section on fatigue, below).

In parallel with this there is a reduction in the speed with which nerves conduct impulses, and, because nerves relaying position sense are involved, old people often experience difficulty in maintaining their balance, especially if acutely displaced (jostled or pushed). Although ageing does interfere with muscle power and balance, a careful search should always be made for neurological disease (Table 6.2).

Loss of articular cartilage is probably a natural consequence of ageing. When it is associated with thickening of the underlying bone and bone formation at the joint margins (osteophytes) osteoarthritis is said to be present (Chapter 7), but it may not be the only locomotor cause of disability in old age (Table 6.3).

The previous paragraphs provide evidence that ageing is almost inevitably associated with some decline in neuromuscular performance. This is relatively minor and rarely if ever interferes with self-

Table 6.2 Neurological causes of immobility in the elderly (see also Chapter 8)

Cerebral lesions	Cerebrovascular accidents
	Parkinson's disease
	Advanced senile dementia
	Cerebral tumours
Mid-brain lesions	Vertebrobasilar insufficiency
Cord lesions	Motor neurone disease
	Cord ischaemia
	B_{12} deficiency
	Cord tumours
	Multiple sclerosis
	Tabes dorsalis (rare)
Peripheral nerve lesions	Neoplastic neuropathy
	Diabetes mellitus
	B_{12} deficiency
	Drugs

Table 6.3 Locomotor causes of immobility in the elderly

Structure	Disorder	
Bones	Osteomalacia	Myeloma
	Paget's disease	Bony secondaries
	Osteoporosis	Fractures
Joints	Osteoarthritis	Vascular necrosis of
	Rheumatoid arthritis	femoral head
	"Charcot" joint	Hallux valgus
	Gout	Pyrophosphate arthropathy
Muscles	Myopathy	Motor neurone disease
	Polymyalgia rheumatica	
	Polymyositis	
Feet	Corns	Ischaemic ulcers
	Abnormal growth of	Deformities of feet (pes
	toenails	cavus, equinovarus etc.)
	(onychogryphosis)	

care capacity, so that someone experiencing difficulty in supporting himself at home is not suffering from old age, but from a disease which is usually age related. This is sometimes curable, often treatable and can always be alleviated. Early identification of the problem is essential if loss of independence is to be avoided. This is only possible if all members of the health care team, including the relatives, exercise a high degree of vigilance and suspicion.

MENTAL FUNCTION

Mental Impairment (Chapter 9)

There is considerable debate on whether or not ageing interferes with mental function. An apparent decline is often due to a communication problem, or a catastrophic change in the social situation, such as bereavement, moving to new accommodation (house or residential home), going into hospital or the family going away. The first essential in dealing with apparent mental frailty is to ensure that the patient is obtaining adequate input by correcting visual or hearing defects. Allowance must be made for speech defects, for incoherence is often related to dysarthria or dysphasia rather than mental impairment. In these conditions, a secondary language sometimes is lost, hence English may be lost in those whose primary language is French or Hindustani. Similarly deaf people will often try and hide their disability from strangers and it is easy to become engaged in a bizarre conversation, unless deafness is suspected. Confusion may be compounded by a wide range of physical disorders.

While there is great individual variation, there is no doubt that some aspects of memory are affected by age, as are some information processing mechanisms (Chapters 2 and 9).

Depression (Cases, 3, 6 and 9)

While, depression is no more common in old age than in younger groups there are differences in the precipitating factors and the course which it follows. Changes in the biochemistry of the brain may be important but physical ill health, bereavement and a deteriorating social background often exert a major influence on the severity of depression.

The pain, disability and deprivation caused by chronic illness is often associated with a depressed affect. Traditional teaching is that antidepressants are only of value where depression is the consequence of an intrinsic change in brain function. Practical experience demonstrates that this is not the case. Many lonely and physically disabled old people who are depressed respond extremely well to appropriate drug therapy.

A wide range of social stresses may contribute to depression. Bereavement (Chapter 15) is discussed elsewhere, but other less dramatic causes of isolation may contribute to depression including the marriage of children, the movement of children to a job in another part of the country or world, or rehousing away from a familiar neighbourhood.

Retirement also may be a time of stress, because within 24 hours a man (or a woman) may lose his workmates, suffer a precipitous fall in income, lose a major source of interest and relinquish the family position of breadwinner. It may seem that useful life has ended and that the individual is now a burden on society, and, although this extreme reaction is relatively uncommon, there is need for the more widespread development of pre-retirement courses (Chapter 4).

There are many less well-defined reasons for elderly people being depressed. Modern society tends to devalue the role of age in industry and recreation. Experience is considered to be less important than vitality and originality and this engenders a sense of inferiority which is accentuated by low incomes and inadequate housing.

Although tricyclic antidepressants are extremely effective in many old people they are responsible for a wide range of side effects. These include drowsiness and confusion, and anticholinergic and antiadrenergic effects, including dry mouth, urinary retention, blurring of vision and postural hypotension. The incidence of these has been reduced by using newer tricyclic agents such as lofepramine or doxepin. Even with these substances it is important to start with a small dose gradually building up to therapeutic amounts. As in other age groups, there usually is a lag period of at least 2 weeks before the patient experiences any benefit.

Serotonin reuptake inhibitors also are extremely effective as antidepressants, and are much less toxic (Case 9). They also may have a more rapid onset of action, though further clinical experience is required to confirm this. A major disadvantage is that they are much more expensive than even the newer tricyclic agents and should be reserved for patients with intolerable side effects, or with a poor response to tricyclics.

If a patient is at serious risk from suicide, fails to respond to antidepressant drugs, or is likely to die from severe inanition, consideration should be given to applying unilateral electroconvulsive therapy. This is extremely effective in old people, and unlikely to cause side effects other than a mild transient memory loss.

POOR NUTRITION (Cases 2, 6, 8 and 10)

There is a progressive decline in the intake of energy and nutrients with increasing age, but this is the consequence of a decline in energy expenditure, and poor nutrition is uncommon in old people living independent lives in their own homes. Exceptions to this are individuals with severe mental or physical incapacity. Those whose mobility is restricted by poor vision or by locomotor or neurological defects have difficulty both shopping and preparing food. It has also been recognised that inadequate mastication, associated with dental neglect or worn dentures, leads to poor nutrition. Chronic diseases such as cardiac failure, chronic obstructive airways disease, Parkinson's disease, thyrotoxicosis or previous gastric surgery suppress appetite, increase metabolism or interfere with gastro-intestinal absorption. It is also well recognised that depression may be associated with profound anorexia, while patients with dementia, particularly Alzheimer's disease, are often emaciated. In the latter, this is, in part, due to inadequate food intake, but there also may be a change in the baseline metabolic state, for, in many, all food given is eaten voraciously and they should be given "second helpings". Living alone or having a low income does not have an adverse effect on nutrition, unless accompanied by ill health, in which case they become important compounding factors.

It has proved extremely difficult to identify the effects of under-nutrition in old people. The obvious effect of protein calorie mal-nutrition is muscle wasting and loss of subcutaneous tissue. The effects of reduced intakes of minerals, vitamins and trace elements are less obvious, and deficiency in a single nutrient often appears to have little effect on overall health. Table 6.4 details the effects which may be associated with specific deficiencies, but these often are difficult to define in individual patients.

The first stage in treating poor nutrition is to identify it. This should be facilitated by general practitioners, as part of their con-tract, offering review to all patients over the age of 75 years. Since there is a close relationship between ill health and poor nutrition, the two should be treated simultaneously (Figure 6.2). Control of cardiac failure, for example, will go a long way to relieving the anorexia and negative protein and energy balance associated with

Table 6.4 Clinical problems associated with vitamin and mineral deficiency in elderly patients

Nutrient	Potential clinical condition	Degree of effect
Thiamine	Cardiac failure	Minor
	Peripheral neuropathy	Minor
	Confusion	Major
Riboflavine	Glossitis/angular stomatitis	Minor
Nicotinic acid	Confusion	Uncertain
	Skin pigmentation	Minor
	Glossitis	Minor
	Diarrhoea	Minor
Pyridoxine	Anaemia	Minor
	Impaired glucose tolerance	Minor
Folic acid	Mental impairment	Minor
	Tongue changes	Uncertain
	Diarrhoea	Minor
Ascorbic acid	Delayed wound healing	Major
	Anaemia	Minor
	Reduced resistance to infection	Uncertain
	Purpura	Minor
Vitamin D	Osteomalacia	Uncertain
Iron	Tiredness and lethargy	Minor
	Koilonychia	Minor
	Glossitis	Major
	Anaemia	Minor
Potassium	Cardiac arrhythmia	Major
	Myopathy	Moderate
	Paralytic ileus	Moderate
	Renal impairment	Minor
Calcium	Bone rarefaction	Moderate
Magnesium	Accentuates effects of potassium and calcium deficiency	Uncertain
Zinc	Delayed wound healing	Major
	Reduced resistance to infection	Uncertain
	Loss of taste	Minor

the condition. Measures to ensure a satisfactory dietary intake must be directed toward the provision and preparation of food. If the family or neighbour are unable or unwilling to do this other steps will have to be taken, such as employing a home help to shop and cook meals, organising meals-on-wheels, taking the patient out to a luncheon club, and, if he can be persuaded to take these, providing food supplements. The effect of these measures must be monitored. Many old people are too polite to refuse meals-on-wheels, but do not actually eat them. Others use supplements to supplement the diet of their pets.

Undernourished elderly patients are at particular risk if they develop an acute illness or suffer major trauma such as a fractured proximal femur. They have inadequate reserves to cope with the severe catabolism which usually accompanies such disorders or the subsequent surgery. The problem is further compounded by the severe anorexia which often accompanies such illness. In these circumstances nutrient solutions should be given through a narrow bore nasogastric tube (enternal feeding). This approach can be life saving, but it should be reserved for patients in whom there is a reasonable chance of returning to a good quality of life. It is inappropriate in patients who clearly are dying, or who have severe dementia.

Patients in institutions also have nutritional problems. Severe physical incapacity may mean that they have difficulty in feeding themselves. The problem is made worse when nurses give priority to finishing meal rounds as quickly as possible, and when all courses of the meal are presented at the same time. It takes a lot of time to feed such disabled patients, or to encourage them to feed themselves. Mealtimes must be carefully planned. The kitchen must produce food that is nutritious, palatable (stronger flavouring may be needed to stimulate failing taste and smell), and suited to the needs of individuals who may have difficulty in masticating or swallowing. As has been indicated in the last chapter, collaboration between dietitian, chef, catering officer, nursing and medical staff is essential.

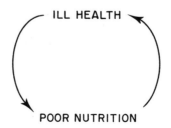

Figure 6.2   Cycle of ill health and poor nutrition

OBESITY

Under-nutrition occurs in a comparatively small proportion of the elderly population. Over-nutrition warrants greater attention. Obesity kills old men, immobilises old women and drives carers to despair. Table 6.5 lists some of its more common complications. The only effective treatment is a reduction of food intake, and because of the inactivity of the elderly this may need to be as low as 600 calories daily, a level which many old people will reject. Increasing activity and thereby energy expenditure will help to increase this level, but weight loss will only be achieved with the patient's active support, convincing him that it is in his interest, by moral support, and gentle bullying from both relatives and health professionals, together with a regular monitoring of his weight. Attending groups such as "Weightwatchers" or special clinics can be often helpful, while day hospitals and day centres can be used to increase activities. Particular attention must be paid to the control of edible gifts from well meaning visitors both at home and in hospital.

FATIGUE

It has long been accepted that decreased physical work capacity is an inevitable consequence of ageing. The older worker, though, can keep up with his younger colleague by taking short-cuts that he has learned through experience, but the reductions in muscle power, in cardiac output and in pulmonary ventilatory capacity are demonstrable in most people. However, recent work suggests that deterioration of many of these processes can be prevented or reversed by carefully graded exercise programmes. It is possible

Table 6.5   Consequences of obesity

Osteoarthritis	Hypertension
Gallbladder disease	Cardiac failure
Hiatus hernia	Accentuated respiratory failure
Reduced carbohydrate tolerance	Immobility and its consequences: venous thrombosis
Coronary artery disease	constipation
Cerebrovascular disease	pressure sores
Peripheral vascular disease	

that the increased expectation of life in the Japanese (Chapter 1) may be due, in part, to this type of organisation of the workplace.

There is no doubt that exercise is a most important factor in promoting health and preventing disability in old people. It was known to Juvenal (A.D 60–130) that soundness of mind and body went together. In his report "On the state of the Public Health for the year 1990" the Chief Medical Officer for England and Wales emphasised that it was important to recognise that old people could benefit from preventive and health promotion programmes. Taking regular physical exercise increases well-being, strength and mobility. This means walking at least one mile a day at as fast a pace as is comfortable. With practice it becomes easier to do and can be done faster. It is important to: begin gradually and increase activity daily; to warm up and warm down; halt activity if it produces any discomfort; avoid sudden twisting and jerking movements and forms of exercise likely to cause falls; avoid outdoor activities in extreme cold or icy conditions; avoid getting overtired. Exercise must be taken regularly, at least three times a week, in order to maintain fitness.

To increase fitness, exercise should involve moderate aerobic activity for about 30 minutes at about 50% of maximum oxygen intake four or five times a week initially, increasing to 60%. The usual maximum oxygen intake for a 65-year-old person, regardless of sex, is 25 to 30 ml/kg/min. Walking at 3.2 km/h (2 m.p.h.) has an oxygen cost of 11; housework has 10; mowing the lawn with a power mower has 14; golf has 14; and dancing—waltzing and square dancing have—14 and 21 respectively.

SKIN CHANGES (Chapter 2)

Decline in the epithelial cell reproduction rate causes thinning of the epidermis and a reduction in sweat glands and sweat secretion. These factors combine to make the skin of old people dry and fragile and a variety of disorders may result.

There may be intolerable itch (pruritus). Changes of temperature induced by undressing, going outdoors or taking a bath may be sufficient to trigger this off. Minor trauma related to woolly underwear may also initiate it and in more severe cases itching may be accompanied by small patches of scaling and redness. The symptom can be controlled by using bath oils (oilatum emollient) and inexpensive cold creams to keep the skin moist, and by avoiding extremes of temperature and rough clothing.

Local changes in the skin and a general reduction in immunological mechanisms increase the susceptibility of old people to skin infections. Fungal and, in particular, monilial infections can be very troublesome, the organism attacking areas of skin already damaged by other factors. Nurses who have difficulty in clearing up a breast intertrigo or urine rash should always consider this possibility and seek medical advice, for treatment with an appropriate antifungal cream will often solve the problem.

Sebaceous dermatitis consists of an itchy, red and scaly rash which starts in the scalp and extends downwards to involve the neck, shoulders and chest. Despite its name, there is doubt as to whether it is really related to an abnormal sebaceous secretion. It can be controlled by regularly washing the scalp with a cleansing agent such as cetrimide (Seboderm).

Ageing causes a reduction of the number of skin pigment cells, which accounts for the greying of the hair and skin pallor found in many old people. Along with an overall decline there may be local areas of pigment cell proliferation. This can produce a striking form of freckling involving exposed surfaces such as the forearm. It is of no clinical significance.

Old people exhibit a diffuse reduction in the density of hair follicles both on the scalp and on the rest of the body. Occasionally, the condition is a result of thyroid or vitamin C deficiency but it is quite distinct from localised hereditary baldness which comes on in middle life in many males.

FURTHER READING

Cullinan, T. (1986). *Visual Disorders in the Elderly*. London: Croom Helm.

DOH (1992). *Report on Health and Social Subjects, No 43. The nutrition of elderly people: Report of the working group on the nutrition of elderly people of the Committee on Medical Aspects of Food Policy*. London: HMSO.

Hinchcliffe, R. (1983). *Hearing and Balance in the Elderly*. London: Churchill Livingstone.

Horwitz, A., MacFadyen, D.M., Munro, H. *et al.*, (1989). *Nutrition in the Elderly*. Oxford: Oxford University Press.

Marks, R. (1987). *Skin Disease in Old Age*. London: Martin Dunitz.

Murphy, E. (1986). *Affective Disorders in the Elderly*. London: Churchill Livingstone.

Shepherd, R.J. (1987). *Physical Activity and Ageing*, (2nd Edn), London: Croom Helm.

CHAPTER 7   The musculoskeletal system

MUSCLES

It is a universal observation that increasing age is associated with a decline in muscle power (Figure 7.1). A major factor in this is muscle atrophy due to the death of progressive numbers of anterior horn cells in the spinal cord, though changes in the motor end plate may precede loss of spinal motor neurones. This process starts early in life, and the longest axons tend to be affected first. The result is a reduction of Type II muscle fibres (fast twitch), but at this stage surviving nerves sprout extra axon branches to reinnervate the recently denervated muscle fibres. Eventually, however, the task becomes too great for the surviving nerves so that in old age there is a striking reduction in power.

This is only part of the story. Another reason for declining strength in old age is reduced physical activity. The old saw "if you don't use it, you lose it" is true and it has been demonstrated graphically in industrial workers that a dramatic decline in thigh muscle mass occurs within a few months of retirement. Diet is also important. Sick old people may not eat sufficient protein to meet muscle requirements and this leads to further muscle wasting (Case 1). The message then is that ageing does produce a decline in strength, but that this can be minimised by indulging in regular exercise, combined with a well-balanced diet.

Myopathies

Despite the effects of ageing, healthy old people should be fully mobile and able to perform all self-care activities. In the absence of joint or neurological disease, an old person who has difficulty in walking or getting out of a chair is likely to be suffering from

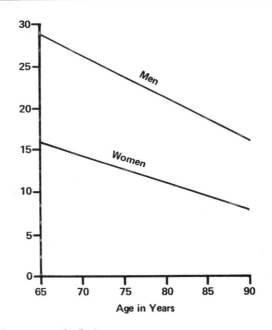

Figure 7.1   Grip strength (kg)

a muscle disease (myopathy). Although inflammatory and toxic myopathies occur in the elderly, and people with muscular dystrophy live into old age, metabolic and endocrine disorders are the commonest causes (Table 7.1) and can usually be treated by dietary replacement or drug manipulation. These measures are likely to be ineffective unless the patient is put onto a rehabiliation programme. In vitamin D deficiency, for example, there is gross weakness of the thigh muscles, so that hip flexion exercises by the physiotherapist, reinforced by the nursing staff encouraging mobilisation, are essential if the patient is to make progress.

Muscle Pain

General

Muscle pain due to unaccustomed exercise, exposure to cold, or psychological stress is common in all age groups, and usually responds to reassurance and treatment with a mild analgesic. The great danger in old age is that patients and sometimes their doctors attribute aches and pains to "rheumatism" or "fibrositis" without adequate investigation, thereby missing serious and often poten-

Table 7.1   Causes of metabolic and endocrine myopathic syndromes

Hyperthyroidism	Hypothyroidism
Hypercalcaemia	Carcinomatosis
Hyperaldosteronism	Vitamin D deficiency
Hypokalaemia	

Drugs: steroids, metolazone, alcohol, H_2 antagonists, antimicrobials, cytotoxic agents

tially treatable underlying disorders, e.g. polymyositis and dermato-myositis.

Polymyalgia rheumatica

This is a disorder characterised by severe pain and stiffness of the shoulder and pelvic girdles, particularly in the early morning. Examination reveals tenderness but not weakness of the affected muscles, and the diagnosis is confirmed by finding a high erythro-cyte sedimentation rate (ESR). The diagnosis is a rewarding one to make in that the patient responds dramatically to steroids and within a matter of days is pain-free and fully mobile.

Another important reason for making the diagnosis is that the condition is often associated with inflammation of the cranial arter-ies (giant cell arteritis). When this happens the temporal artery is commonly affected (temporal arteritis) and feels tender and swollen. If the occipital arteries are involved the scalp over them may be tender. Sometimes these signs are missing. If the retinal or cerebral arteries are involved the patient may suffer sudden loss of vision in one eye or develop a stroke. Steroid therapy is effective in controlling the condition and preventing complications. Biopsy of the temporal artery should be performed in all cases in which the diagnosis is suspected.

The starting dose of steroids should be high, say 45 mg of predni-solone daily, in divided doses. Once symptoms have settled, and once the ESR has begun to fall, the dose may be reduced gradually to the lowest level which maintains a normal ESR and keeps the patient symptom free. Usually a maintenance level of 5 or 10 mg is achieved. If the ESR has remained within the normal range for about 3 months, then steroids can be gradually withdrawn. It is wise to monitor the ESR for a period after steroids have been stopped, and restart treatment if the ESR rises or the patient com-plains of a return of symptoms. If a diagnosis of temporal arteritis has been confirmed, it may be necessary to continue treatment for a much longer period of time, and some patients may need to continue for years, requiring a maintenance dose of prednisolone as high as 20 mg daily. This is likely to be associated with a wide range of side effects.

Muscle Cramps

Muscle cramps are common and often quite disabling. They tend to occur during the night and may be so disturbing as to cause severe depression, occasionally leading to suicide. The cause is not always obvious and in the majority of patients none can be found. Cramps may be associated with vitamin deficiency, uraemia, hypo-kalaemia, peripheral vascular disease or neurological disability. The drugs used to try to ameliorate this condition are legion. More than one may need to be tried before success is achieved. Quinine sulphate and diazepam are probably the most successful, although often the only relief is to get up and make a cup of tea; another remedy is to raise the head of the bed on blocks of wood. If these measures are unsuccessful, anticonvulsants, antidepressants and vasodilators may be tried. (Epilepsy in the elderly can present as attacks of unilateral pain without convulsions—Chapter 8.) It should be remembered that all the drugs mentioned are potentially hazardous. Therefore before any of these are prescribed the severity of this symptom and the distress it is causing must be carefully assessed. In particular, quinine may be responsible for hearing and visual disturbances, a blotchy skin rash, and, rarely, thrombocytopenia.

JOINT DISEASE

Ageing of Joints

Articular cartilage, especially that involved in weight-bearing joints, undergoes changes throughout life from about the age of 25 years onwards. The material becomes more opaque, firmer and yellowish in colour, is less elastic and more resistant to deformation. Though cartilage is capable of repairing itself this ability diminishes with ageing. Cartilage consists, almost entirely, of collagen Type II with an interfibrillary matrix of proteoglycans linked to hyaluronic acid. Proteolytic enzymes from chondrocytes continually break down this matrix and synthetise new matrix. With ageing there is reduction in size of the proteoglycan molecules, more of which remain unbound to hyaluronic acid with an increase in the concentration of hyaluronic acid and reduction in water. The synovial membrane becomes denser and thickened with villous hypertrophy. Sclerosis and occlusion of capsular arterioles leading to local vascular insufficiency is associated with these changes.

Osteoarthritis (Cases 6, 7 and 10)

The notion that this occurs solely as the result of "wear and tear" is old-fashioned. The condition is common in old people and is characterised by loss of articular cartilage, thickening of the underlying bone surfaces and expansion of bone around the edges of the joint (osteophyte formation). Biochemically, there is a reduction in the proteoglycan content of the cartilage, but increased synthesis, with changes in the structure of the proteoglycan molecules and a marked increase in the water content of the cartilage. While the aetiology is uncertain there is clear evidence that the condition is associated with trauma, inflammation, biochemical changes and genetic influences. Some of the commoner causes are listed in Table 7.2.

The condition can affect any joint. The symptoms are those of stiffness and pain. Movement increases the pain which leads to immobility. It usually starts in a single joint and then tends to spread to others. The onset is usually insiduous but it may be acute. It may occur at any time from middle age onwards. Some women develop an acute form affecting the proximal and distal phalangeal joints (Bouchard's and Heberden's nodes) which become swollen, painful and unsightly, though they later become pain free. This often occurs just after the menopause.

Table 7.2   Conditions predisposing to osteoarthritis

Obesity	Rheumatoid arthritis
Trauma	Gout
Old infection	Steroids
Developmental changes (e.g. Perthes' disease)	Paget's disease

Hips and knees (Case 7)

The disease causes most pain and disability if these large joints are affected. Flexion and extension of the knee is painful, and may be accompanied by a grating sensation (crepitus), which can be felt. The bony deformation of the knee prevents hyperextension during weight-bearing and the locking mechanism is therefore lost. Thus the leg is always at risk of unexpectedly "giving way" causing the patient to fall. The diagnosis of hip involvement may be more diffcult for pain is sometimes referred to the knee. Hip flexion, again, may be normal and pain only produced by external and internal rotation.

Treatment should aim at controlling pain and improving mobility. The simplest analgesic should be used in the first instance. Paracetamol given in divided doses regularly throughout the day up to a total of 4 g is very effective. Alternatively one of the many non-steroidal anti-inflammatory drugs may be used. The simplest of these is a buffered aspirin, or ibuprofen which combines efficacy with safety. It must be remembered that all this group of drugs have side effects and have been particularly associated with gastro-intestinal bleeding, renal damage and fluid retention (Case 7). Patients should be warned to report symptoms of indigestion, but gastric irritation and bleeding may be symptomless, so it is wise to keep the haemoglobin concentration under review. Local treatment such as ice, heat or diathermy produces temporary alleviation of discomfort, but little long-term benefit. If these methods fail then intra-articular injection of steroids may be useful. The injection is likely to be more effective if the patient has a tender spot which can be injected. Repeated injection is not justifiable, and can lead to serious destruction of the articular surfaces (Charcot's joint).

The physiotherapist has an important part to play in the management of these patients. Active and passive movements help to maintain muscle strength and maintain mobility. Relatives and nursing staff should back this up by encouraging the patient to walk rather than be wheeled or carried during day-to-day activities. If he is obese the help of the dietitian should be enlisted to achieve weight loss. The day hospital has a very useful part to play in the management of many elderly patients with osteoarthritis, for not only can diagnosis be confirmed but treatment deployed and an overall strategy worked out to achieve and maintain optimum function of the patient in his home surroundings (Chapter 5).

Joint replacement

Where osteoarthritis is particularly crippling, surgery should be considered. Total hip (Case 5) and knee replacement with a prosthesis is very effective. There is almost no person who is too old for surgery (Chapter 5). For the operation to be a success, however, the patient must want to have the operation, be fit enough to tolerate the procedure and have sufficient mental drive and ability to collaborate with the rehabilitation programme afterwards. Orthopaedic surgeons are now so skilled and prostheses so good that there is almost no joint that cannot be successfully replaced. Close collaboration between the orthopaedic surgeon and the geriatrician is most important.

Vertebral column (Case 6)

Degeneration of connective tissue in the vertebral discs, and destruction of cartilage in the posterior (apophyseal) joints conspire to produce severe back pain in old age. However, back pain is a common complaint, and diagnoses, other than that of osteoarthritis, must be excluded before treatment is organised. Table 7.3 lists possible causes which should be considered. Evidence of root compression, such as sciatica, should always be sought. An insidious form of nerve compression is that involving the cauda equina, causing incontinence of urine and faeces and numbness of the buttocks leading to the development of pressures sores. If surgical treatment is to be successful then the condition must be identified at an early stage, when the patient only complains of pain in the buttocks while walking.

Where the dorsal and lumbar vertebrae are involved, treatment with analgesics should be coupled with advice on sleeping on a firmer mattress, and exercises designed to increase local mobility and relieve spasm (Table 7.4). If the patient does not have a firm

Table 7.3   Causes of back pain

Muscle trauma	Multiple myeloma
Osteoarthritis	Tuberculosis
Prolapsed disc	Gastric disease
Vertebral trauma	Pancreatic disease
Osteoporosis/osteodystrophy	Renal disease
Secondary cancer	Herpes zoster

mattress, placing wooden boards under the patient's mattress is sufficient to achieve a firm base on which to sleep. Surgical corsets are best avoided in that they result in muscle wasting, are difficult to put on, and thus tend to increase dependence.

Osteoarthritis in the neck (cervical spondylosis) (Case 6) presents a more complex problem since, in addition to causing neck pain, it may be associated with spinal cord compression, nipping of nerve roots and compression of the vertebral arteries. A popular remedy is a cervical collar, but this tends to be loose fitting and useless, or well fitting and uncomfortable. If pain is very severe a well fitted Plastozote collar may be helpful in the short term. Otherwise simple analgesics or, in more severe cases, a non-steroidal anti-inflammatory drug should be given. In patients with very severe pain or early, progressive neurological signs surgical fixation may be indicated. Usually symptoms can be prevented and/or relieved if the patient pays attention to his posture and performs simple neck exercises (Table 7.4).

Damage to the apophyseal joints interferes with the function of mechanoreceptors sited there. This results in the mid-brain and medulla being supplied with inadequate information on the position of the neck, so that the patient experiences symptoms of vertigo, unsteadiness and dizziness. Balance may also be impaired by the direct compression of the spinal cord from osteophytes around the vertebral disc. Again, falls may be the result of brain stem ischaemia associated with compression of the vertebral arteries by osteophytes. There is increasing evidence, however, that these last two conditions are relatively rare causes of dizziness and unsteadiness, and that even the apparently classic picture of ver-

Table 7.4   General exercises for the osteoarthritic elderly patient whose intervertebral joints are involved

---

1. Slump down in chair. Go limp, then straighten spine to full (sitting) height slowly.
   Repeat three or four times.

2. Rock forward toward toes. Lift leg with bent knee from the ground for a count of 5 then lower slowly, alternate legs. Slap feet on floor, first slowly then more quickly.

3. Press right then left arm alternately on chair arms, taking as much weight as possible.

4. Shrug shoulders up to ears several times. Rotate head slowly right and left several times.

---

tigo associated with sudden movements of the neck is more likely to be the result of the mechano-receptor degeneration than of either cord compression or vertebral artery stenosis.

Shoulder Movement

Diminished shoulder movement may occur as the result of osteoarthritic changes, but when only a single joint is involved, it is more usually due to inflammation of the joint capsule. This most commonly occurs after a stroke when, in the early stages, loss of support from muscles of the shoulder puts excessive strain on joint ligaments. It is best avoided by ensuring after a stroke that at all times the arm and forearm are supported. At the same time, passive and active exercises should be employed to keep the joint mobile. Once developed, the condition should be treated with local exercise, but often it proves extremely refactory to treatment. Local injections of hydrocortisone may occasionally help.

As in other age groups damage to structures around the shoulder, such as the long head of biceps, subacromial bursa or infraspinatus tendon, may give rise to a painful arc syndrome in which adduction of the joint is limited to about 30 degrees. Local treatment with heat or diathermy or injection of the target with corticosteroids may be helpful.

Rheumatoid Arthritis

Rheumatoid arthritis is common in the elderly population affecting 2% of men and 5.5% of women over 65 years. While new cases may occur, it has often been present a long time, since youth or middle age. It may be associated with severe deformity such as subluxation of the metacarpophalangeal joints, fixed shoulders, flexion deformities of knees, gross deformity of the feet and dislocation of the atlanto-axial joint. This type of patient is often referred to the geriatrician for long-term care, since his continuing care at home is proving impossible. Often this situation has arisen because of inadequate or inappropriate treatment or because the patient has rejected the advice and treatment prescribed. Fortunately advances in the field of rheumatology and better services have made this type of patient less common. In particular, early operative treatment and modern prosthetics have meant that it has been possible to correct and prevent deformity by replacing joints and freeing tendons (synovectomy) involved in the disease process.

The very disabled patient presents a major challenge to the therapeutic team and it is most important to consider the whole patient, his environment and his support system. The occupational therapist and the physiotherapist must collaborate to maximise function; the doctor and the nurse must monitor the response to drug treatment, and the patient's morale and assess his pootential quality of life; relatives, social workers and volunteers must help to provide variety, and plan for the future, thereby giving the patient hope. It has to be remembered that the patient is likely to be well versed in medical lore and to have experienced much failure. Optimism is essential but must be tempered with reality. In the intelligent patient, gadgetry ranging from lazy tongs to an electric wheelchair or to a Possum can make a major difference to quality of life. No possible remedy should be discarded without careful consideration and consultation with the patient.

Rheumatoid arthritis developing for the first time in an elderly patient may present abruptly as an acute illness. Joint pain (arthralgia) and muscle pain (myalgia) may be severe and accompanied by systemic effects such as pyrexia, nausea and rigors. The diagnosis is confirmed by a high ESR and positive serological tests for rheumatoid factor. Despite the dramatic onset, the prognosis is often quite good and the patient may be relatively asymptomatic after a period of one or two years. Late onset rheumatoid has a lower incidence of extra-articular features.

Drug treatment of rheumatoid arthritis is essentially that of any age, but the drug side effects increasingly dominate the picture. Examples include tinnitus and blood loss with salicylates and other non-steroidal anti-inflammatory (NSAI) drugs, albuminuria and evidence of renal damage with gold (reversible if drug discontinued), and osteoporosis and broken bones with corticosteroids. For similar reasons, penicillamine or immunosuppressant drugs should be used with caution in older patients.

The therapeutic strategy varies with the prejudices of the clinician, but a reasonable approach might be to start with standard dose of ibuprofen, and, where this fails, try another non-steroidal anti-inflammatory agent. If this proves ineffective, second line therapy should be considered. Gold has been used for many years but was out of favour for a time. Now, as sodium aurothiomalate, it is once more proving effective in some patients. It can be given orally or by injection. Side effects such as skin rashes, proteinuria, or marrow failure can be minimised by careful monitoring. Alternatives are penicillamine and sulphasalazine, which have similar efficacy, and anti-malarials, which are less toxic but less effective. Corticosteroids may be used in high dosage for a short course to produce remission but tailed off and stopped as soon as possible. In some elderly, such as those with low life expectancy, it may be justifiable to continue them for an indefinite period. If all these fail the use of a cytotoxic agent such as methotrexate might be considered.

Gout and Pseudogout

Over 10% of patients with gout experience their first attack after they have reached the age of 60 years. Like those who have experienced an attack earlier in life, some have a positive family history. In women, however, and in men with no family history a cause should be sought. Conditions such as the blood dyscrasias, which increase purine metabolism, or renal disease, which reduces the excretion of uric acid, may underlie the onset of an attack. Similarly the chronic intake of alcohol reduces renal excretion of uric acid and explains that characteristic cartoon of the old man with a red nose and a bandaged foot resting on a cushion. With an ageing female population, gout is common in the 90-year-old, particularly if she has been on long-term diuretic therapy. Large doses of an NSAI agent, such as naproxen, should be used to control an acute attack. Thereafter, drugs such as allopurinol and probenecid should be used to maintain serum uric acid levels within normal limits. Both are well tolerated. Treatment should be aimed also at controlling any underlying condition and stopping offending medication.

Pseudogout (pyrophosphate arthropathy) has a similar clinical presentation to classical gout but occurs more commonly in the elderly. The condition results from the formation of pyrophosphate crystals in the synovial fluid. It affects larger joints, in particular the knee, where it can be diagnosed radiologically by characteristic calcification of the semi-lunar cartilages. Treatment and management are as for classical gout, although knee aspiration may abort an attack in the acute phase if swelling occurs. Patients with pseudogout should be investigated to exclude other diseases such as hyperparathyroidism or haemochromatosis.

Miscellaneous

Abnormal pain free joints may be associated with neurological diseases such as diabetic neuropathy, syringomyelia or tabes dorsalis (Charcot's joint), and also may result from the local treatment of a joint with intra-articular injections of steroid, or parenteral treatment with steroid agents. The joints are usually grossly deformed and enlarged, due to bony deformity as well as the effusion of fluid; instability may result and operation may be required to remedy this.

Infective arthritis is also common and although infection usually affects joints which already have been damaged by rheumatoid disease or osteoathritis, normal joints may sometimes be involved. The condition may remain unsuspected if ageing, concurrent disease or treatment with immunosuppressant drugs has suppressed a localised and/or systemic inflammatory response to infection. Alternatively the only manifestation may be the systemic effects of septicaemia and, hence, in elderly patients presenting with systemic infections, joint infection should be excluded. The usual infecting organisms are *Staphylococcus*, *Streptococcus*, and *Escherichia*. Steroid therapy, given either systemically or by local injection, often predisposes to the development of the condition.

FEET

Any assessment of the locomotor system should include a careful examination of the feet. Painful feet can severely interfere with mobility and lead to a progressive decline in physical capacity. Table 7.5 lists some of the more common conditions to be identified. Many of these problems require the skilled attention of a chiropodist or even an orthopaedic surgeon, but simple measures such as advice on footwear, or help in clipping nails, may be all that is required.

Table 7.5 Common foot problems in the elderly

Corns	Peripheral ischaemia
Hammer toes	Trophic ulcer
Hallux valgus	Onychogryphosis
Bunions	(thickened nail)
Plantar wart	Fungal infection

BONES

Bone Ageing and Osteoporosis

Bone mass increases rapidly throughout adolescence followed by a more gradual continuous increment ending between the age of 30 and 40 years. Men by virtue of their greater height and weight end up with a greater bone mass than women. Other factors increasing maximal bone mass are a high level of physical activity, and a reasonable level of dietary calcium in childhood and adolescence.

Bone mass remains stable in women until after the menopause when, for several years, there is a rapid loss of bone mass. This follows oestrogen deficiency in which there is reduced calcitonin secretion, leading to bone resorption and a negative calcium balance. After a few years the bone loss is less severe but continues indefinitely for the rest of life. Men experience less profound loss in old age. This is thought to be due to changes in androgen metabolism, though the precise mechanism remains far from clear.

Factors which exacerbate bone loss include a premature menopause resulting from oophorectomy, immobility associated with chronic ill health and treatment with corticosteroids. A variety of diseases including thyrotoxicosis, rheumatoid arthritis, previous partial gastrectomy and chronic renal failure also are associated with a reduced bone mass.

The end point of continued bone loss is osteoporosis, a situation in which the mechanical strength of bone is reduced to the extent that a patient sustains fractures. Such fractures follow an interesting epidemiological pattern with fractures of the wrist predominating in women in the immediate postmenopausal period, in part associated with a marked deterioration of balance which occurs at the same time. Over the age of 70 years fractures of the proximal femur become increasingly common, presumably because old people have insufficient reflexes to protect themselves from falling on an outstretched arm.

With advancing years spontaneous fractures of the vertebral bodies become increasingly common. These manifest themselves as recurrent episodes of severe localised back pain and kyphosis of the dorsal spine. This is sometimes of such severity that the chest is squeezed into the pelvis and the patient experiences considerable discomfort. Respiratory function may also be compromised, and changes in the centre of gravity have an adverse effect upon mobility.

Osteoporosis is diagnosed by demonstrating bone rarefaction on an X-ray. In the spine, there is concavity of the adjacent surfaces of the vertebral bodies, and anterior wedging of bodies in which there has been a fracture. The serum calcium, phosphate and alkaline phosphatase concentrations usually are normal, though the latter may be elevated if there has been a recent fracture.

The best way of managing osteoporosis is to prevent it. This should start early in life by encouraging everyone to take regular exercise. Most individuals in Western Europe and the United States have intakes of calcium which are more than adequate, but in some parts of East Asia dietary counselling may be necessary to correct calcium deficiency associated with a high incidence of fractures in later life. There is debate as to whether calcium supplementation is useful after the menopause. Large doses reduce the rate of bone loss, but the effect is less striking than that associated with other preventative measures.

The most popular method of reducing postmenopausal bone loss is oestrogen (hormone) replacement therapy (HRT). Concern has been expressed about the effects of this on the incidence of carcinoma of the breast and uterus, but this is not a problem so long as the dose of oestrogen is kept low and it is given cyclically in combination with a progestagen. Concerns about its effect on the incidence of stroke and coronary artery disease have also been unfounded. The difficulty is in deciding which women should be treated. Women at particular risk of osteoporosis include those who are small, thin, have had an early menopause or have a family history of the condition. Attempts have been made to develop biochemical and radiological markers, but these do not have sufficient specificity for them to be of use in routine clinical practice.

Etidronate disodium, an oral bisphosphonate, inhibits osteoclastic activity thus reducing bone resorption. Studies have shown that in women with postmenopausal osteoporosis, intermittent cyclical therapy with etidronate increases spinal bone mass and significantly reduces the incidence of new vertebral fractures. The effectiveness seems to be highest in those patients with most bone loss. It is likely that etidronate will replace other forms of treatment because it is so free of side effects in long-term use.

Osteomalacia

Adults with inadequate amounts of vitamin D develop osteo-malacia, a condition in which there is softening of bone due to inadequate calcification of its protein matrix (osteoid). It is a particular problem in housebound old people. A low exposure to ultra-violet radiation in sunlight reduces the synthesis of vitamin D from cutaneous 7-dehydrocholesterol.

The condition is associated with painful bones and a proximal myopathy which causes a characteristic waddling gait. Softening of bones produces deformities of the thorax and spinal column similar to those found in osteoporosis. Some patients with osteomalacia sustain a fractured proximal femur, but, in most instances, the fracture is due to coincidental osteoporosis.

Investigation reveals low serum calcium and phosphate and high alkaline phosphatase concentrations. A characteristic radiological change is that of narrow bands of radiolucency at right angles to cortical surfaces (Looser's zones). These are not always present and the only abnormality may be reduced bone density and vertebral wedge fractures similar to those found in osteoporosis.

Treatment is with vitamin D. A single injection of 15 mg of calciferol is sufficient to provide adequate amounts of vitamin D for more than 6 months. It is wise to combine this with daily supplements of calcium to ensure that treatment does not increase serum calcium levels at the expense of further skeletal calcification. A disadvantage of giving regular doses of vitamin D orally is that there may be problems of compliance and that overdosage may result in hypercalcaemia with all its attendant side effects.

Paget's Disease

Paget's disease of bone is characterised by an increase in the rate of bone turnover accompanied by remodelling of the bone contour. Its incidence rises with increasing age, and it currently affects three quarters of a million people in Britain. The majority have no symptoms, and it is often only recognised following radiology for some other purpose. Nevertheless, 5% have considerable disability. The cause is as yet unknown, but recently a viral aetiology has been proposed and the canine distemper virus suggested as a possibility. However, this should be viewed with caution.

The condition is important since it may be associated with

symptoms which arise from complications (Table 7.6). The most important of these are bone pain, deafness, fractures, heart failure and malignant change (2% of cases).

Bisphosphonates and calcitonin are the two most effective agents. Both substances reduce urinary hydroxyproline and serum alkaline phosphatase concentrations, by diminishing bone resorption and as a result decreasing bone turnover. Pain is relieved thereby and fractures may heal faster, while spinal cord and nerve compression may be halted and possibly reversed. The bisphosphonate most commonly used is etidronate disodium. It is given in a dose of 5mg/kg/day by mouth for a period of about 6 months. Regression of symptoms may last for a considerable time after a course of treatment. New bisphosphonates, such as pamidronate, are currently undergoing trials, and the suppression of Paget's disease may be a realistic goal in the near future. Calcitonin, which has to be given by injection and may produce unpleasant side effects (headaches and flushing), may then be needed no longer.

Fractured Proximal Femur

In old age there is a geometrical rise in the incidence of fractures of the proximal end of the femur (Figure 7.2). This partly results from the high prevalence of disorders such as osteoporosis, osteomalacia and Paget's disease. Equally important is the increased risk of old people falling (Chapter 8). Recognition of this risk and preventing falls is one way of reducing the incidence of fractures. Patients with fractures are more likely to be demented, to have poor vision, to have cerebrovascular disease or to suffer from drop attacks. General principles in the management of the condition include the following:

Table 7.6 Complications of Paget's disease of bone

Bone pain
Joint deformity → osteoarthritis
Platybasia → deafness
Paraplegia
Cranial nerve compression
High output cardiac failure
Osteogenic sarcoma
Fractures

1. Surgical intervention is essential. Treatment with traction is useless, as it invariably produces permanent immobility in old people.
2. Patients should be thoroughly investigated for intercurrent medical disorders. An old lady will not get better if her cardiac failure, anaemia or diabetes remain untreated.
3. Secondary causes of the fracture should be excluded. Osteomalacia, metastatic deposits and Paget's disease will modify the surgical management.
4. A multidisciplinary rehabilitation programme should be organised (Chapter 5).

Usually the fracture is an episode in a long period of illness associated with multiple pathology and physical incapacity. It is obvious that the geriatrician must be involved in the management of the patient from the outset and that there should be close liaison with the medical, nursing and rehabilitation staff of the orthopaedic unit. A high proportion of patients require prolonged

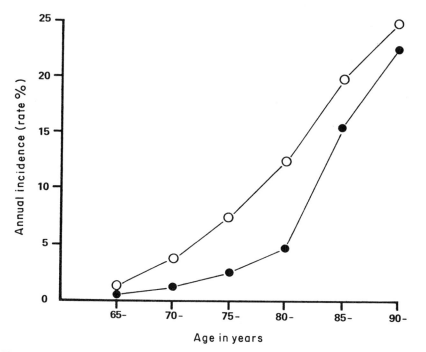

Figure 7.2 Incidence of fractured proximal neck of femur in men ● and women ○ (After Grimley Evans, 1979, *Age and Ageing*, 8, 16–23, with permission)

rehabilitation, and need to be transferred to an orthogeriatric ward run under the joint supervision of a geriatrician and orthopaedic surgeon. Even after discharge, follow-up by a nurse skilled in the management of elderly patients with orthopaedic problems may be useful. Figure 7.3 outlines the system operating currently in Edinburgh.

Fractured Wrist

Fractures of the distal radius and ulna reach their peak incidence in women immediately after the menopause, but remain common in old age. While in youth, a broken wrist is painful and unpleasant, the situation in old age is often complicated by the patient already being disabled in other ways, and living either alone or with a frail and elderly spouse or sibling. Major problems can arise if such a patient is then sent off home. Before this happens the general practitioner and social services department should be alerted so that appropriate services such as a district nurse, a home

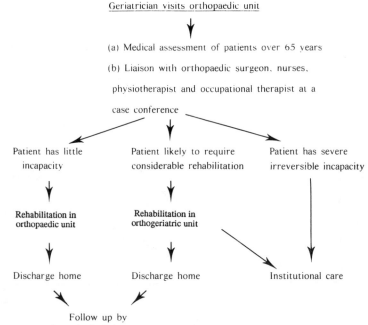

Figure 7.3 Flow chart for management of elderly patients with severe trauma

help or visits from neighbours can be organised. In extreme situations, indeed, it may be necessary to admit the patient to hospital and, ideally, provision for this should be available within the geriatric service.

Fractures of the Vertebrae and Ribs

In old people bone rarefaction may be so severe that seemingly trivial injuries may result in a collapsed vertebral body or a fractured rib. Indeed, even a cough, a yawn or a hearty laugh may do a surprising amount of damage.

When treating a collapsed vertebral body a balance must be struck between providing sufficient rest to relieve pain, and maintaining sufficient mobility to prevent further decalcification and to arrest deterioration in general function. Management of this injury, therefore, calls for close liaison between doctors, nurses and physiotherapists.

Where ribs are fractured the great danger is that a reduction in respiratory excursion will result in a chest infection and pneumonia. Strapping, therefore, should be avoided wherever possible. Sufficient analgesia must be given to relieve pain, so that the patient can take deep breaths, yet oversedation must be avoided, so that respiration is unimpaired. Injection of local anaesthetics is often beneficial. The physiotherapist has an important role in encouraging the maximum use of the thorax despite the considerable amount of discomfort involved in doing so.

Frequently, collapsed vertebrae or broken ribs are due to the blood-borne spread of tumour cells, and in this situation treatment with radiotherapy, cytotoxic drugs or hormones may have to be considered (Chapter 15).

FURTHER READING

Hiskins, D.W. and Nelson M.A. (1987). *The Ageing Spine*. Manchester: Manchester University Press.

MacLennan, W.J. (1990). *Giant cell (temporal) arteritis and polymyalgia*. In *Merck Manual of Geriatrics* (eds. W.B. Abrams and R. Berkow). Merck Sharp & Dohme: pp. 703–710.

Newman, R.J. (1991). *Orthogeriatrics*. London: Butterworth-Heinemann.

Woolf, A.D. and Dixon, A.St.J. (1988). *Osteoporosis—A Clinical Guide*. London: Martin Dunitz.

Wright, V. (1983). *Bone and Joint Disease in the Elderly*. Chichester: Wiley.

CHAPTER 8   The neurology of old age

The physician practising geriatric medicine spends a lot of time dealing with the ravages of neurological disease, often being asked to see the patient when "nothing more can be done". In some instances, modern drug treatment has made it possible to use simple measures to revolutionise the life of the patient. In others, such as cerebrovascular disease, the path to improvement is harder and longer. Nonetheless, attention to detail in diagnosis and assessment, and the use of positive and modern rehabilitation techniques usually pay long-term dividends in terms of mobility, self-sufficiency and self-respect.

STROKE ILLNESS

A stroke is a focal disturbance of brain function related to blockage of, or haemorrhage from, an artery supplying an area of the cerebral hemispheres or brain stem. Manifestations range from transient limb weakness or visual impairment (transient ischaemic attack), through permanent unilateral paralysis with severe sensory disturbance, to deep coma and depression of vital centres.

Aetiology

A variety of factors increase the risk of cerebral thrombosis or haemorrhage. The most important of these is hypertension. Most longitudinal studies have established that, in men and women under the age of 85 years, a blood pressure in excess of 160/90 mmHg is associated with an increased morbidity and mortality from cerebrovascular disease. Patients with diabetes mellitus (IDDM or NIDDM, see Chapter 13) also are at increased risk. Cigarette smoking increases the risk of cerebral thrombosis. While a moderate consumption of alcohol may have a beneficial effect upon the vascular system, heavy drinking increases the risk of stroke.

Information on risk factors has been of great importance in developing measures for the prevention of stroke. Thus a recent reduction in the incidence of the disease in the United States has been the result of more effective control of hypertension, and a reduction in the number of smokers.

Stroke may occasionally be the consequence of an arteritis. In old age the most common type is giant cell arteritis (Chapter 7), but arterial damage associated with systemic lupus erythematosus or polyarteritis nodosa is encountered occasionally.

Clinical Presentation

Transient ischaemic neurological attack (TIA)

This is defined as a focal neurological deficit associated with vascular disease which resolves within 24 hours. Signs include monocular blindness, limb weakness, diplopia, dizziness, dysphasia or sensory disturbance. The condition usually is due to platelet microemboli, and a search should be made for the source of these. More common sites are the bifurcation of the carotid artery, the ostium of the vertebral artery, and damaged mitral and aortic valves. Ophthalmoscopy sometimes reveals platelet fragments within the retinal blood vessels. Less common causes of transient ischaemic attacks are hypertension and paroxysmal cardiac arrhythmias.

A large proportion of patients with attacks associated with carotid artery stenosis eventually sustain a full blown stroke. The course of patients with vertebral artery disease is much more benign, and symptoms often resolve spontaneously.

Completed stroke (Case 3)

A number of clinical rating scales have been developed to distinguish between cerebral thrombosis and haemorrhage, but these have insufficient specificity for them to be reliable in the management of individual patients. If the distinction is of clinical importance, computerised tomography is essential. This normally should be delayed for 3 days, since it takes this time for the evolution of radiological signs of ischaemia.

Systemic embolism must always be excluded as a cause of stroke. The usual causes are mitral valve disease and atrial fibrillation. The latter is such a common condition in old age, however, that the occurrence of atrial fibrillation and stroke does not always represent cause and effect.

Consideration also should be given to conditions other than vascular disease as causes of focal cerebral signs. The most important of these is a benign or malignant cerebral tumour. A useful guide is the rate of onset, in that vascular signs develop relatively quickly, if not instantaneously, over a period of minutes or hours, whereas those associated with a tumour usually take days or weeks. Symptoms and signs of increased intracranial pressure such as headache, vomiting and papilloedema are uncommon in old people. This is due to the fact that the tumour often develops in the presence of coincidental cerebral atrophy. Investigation should consist of looking for evidence of primary tumour such as a bronchial carcinoma, and making a definitive diagnosis by computed tomography.

If a patient is found lying on the ground it can be difficult to decide whether focal neurological signs are the result of the accident or whether they were already present. Features of a subdural haemorrhage include fluctuating signs of drowsiness, clouding of consciousness and confusion. Sometimes, however, these features are less prominent, and there are more focal neurological abnormalities. If there is any doubt about the diagnosis, computerised tomography should be instigated. Any delay may be fatal, or, at best, result in a permanent neurological deficit.

Much less common causes of a hemiparesis are encephalomyelitis, neurosyphilis and bacterial or tuberculous meningitis. These should only be considered if there are convincing clinical features to support such unusual diagnoses.

Assessment of Impairment

Once the diagnosis of a stroke and its cause has been established, and appropriate treatment organised, attention should be directed to assessing the effect of this on neurological function. This is essential if the correct programme of rehabilitation is to be prescribed. Details of this should also be recorded in a systematic fashion so that the progress of the patient and his response to therapy can be charted accurately.

Table 8.1   Changes in function after a stroke

Mental impairment	Apraxia
Depression	Loss of position sense
Emotional lability	Astereognosis
Dysphasia	Agnosia
Dysarthria	Homonymous hemianopia
Dysphagia	Neglect of affected side
Muscle weakness	Denial of illness
Changed muscle tone	Changed bladder tonus

A preliminary is to establish the premorbid condition. Disorders such as dementia (Chapter 9), osteoarthritis (Chapter 7) or cardiorespiratory disease (Chapters 10 and 11) limit the extent to which a patient can cooperate and benefit from a rehabilitation programme.

A detailed evaluation should then be made of his present neurological status. The changes that may occur are listed in Table 8.1. The most important of these relates to cognitive ability. If this is impaired it will be extremely difficult to retrain the patient. Progress often is compromised by depression, and this must be identified and treated. A distinction should be made between depression and emotional lability which is a common feature of stroke illness. Explanation of the condition and encouragement go a long way to limiting the adverse effects of this embarrassing state.

Muscle power should be assessed (Table 8.2) as should muscle tone. Contrary to popular conception, muscles are usually flaccid immediately after a stroke, and it may take several weeks for them to become spastic. Modern physiotherapy techniques mean that patients are far less likely to develop severe spasticity and contractures.

The patient may present with a motor aphasia in which he is unable to find words for particular objects or concepts, a fluid

Table 8.2   Grades used in assessing recovery of muscle power

Complete paralysis	0
Flicker of movement	1
Movement when gravity removed	2
Movement against gravity	3
Movement weak against resistance	4
Normal compared to unaffected side	5

aphasia in which he speaks in jargon and is unaware that he is doing so, or a perceptive aphasia in which he is unable to follow conversation of others. Aphasia has to be distinguished from dysarthria in which the defect is weakness or apraxia of the muscles of articulation. Closely associated with dysarthria is dysphagia. The more severe forms of this are easily identified, but recent research has revealed that a large proportion of stroke patients retain food in the pyriform fossa, and that this is an important cause of aspiration and recurrent episodes of bronchpneumonia. If there is any suspicion of this the patient should be referred for cine-fluoroscopy.

Damage to the occipital cortex may cause a homonymous hemianopia in which there is loss of vision to one side so that the patient walks into obstructions. A more subtle abnormality is visual neglect in which a patient sees an object but pays no attention to it, and has difficulty reading across a page.

Sensory abnormalities are easily missed, but seriously interfere with rehabilitation. Examples are that if position sense is impaired, a patient will be unable to position his leg properly when walking, or, less seriously, if his appreciation of depth is impaired (astereognosis) he will be unable to manage small change. A more bizarre disorder is agnosia in which he does not recognise the function of objects so that he has difficulty selecting cutlery, using writing materials or selecting the correct item of clothing. He may be unable to fit the sequence of movements together (apraxia) so that he has difficulty dressing, and stays rooted to the spot when he attempts to walk. An even more bizarre sensation is failure to recognise paralysis, failure to identify one side as part of himself or total neglect of one side. In a variant of this there is complete neglect of the environment on the affected side. A visitor approaching from this direction is ignored, but is recognised immediately when he moves to the other side. It is extremely difficult for the patient to describe such disorders, and when he fails to respond to inappropriate treatment he is all too easily labelled as being stupid, lazy or poorly motivated.

Once treatment is started, its efficacy should be evaluated regularly using a simple measure of disability (Table 8.3). If, over several weeks, there has been little change, consideration should be given to modifying the rehabilitation programme or resetting targets for outcome. For example, it may emerge that a patient has poor standing balance, and a more realistic objective may be to make him able to transfer without help, and move around the house by wheelchair.

Management of the Acute Phase

Stroke is a common cause of death in old people. As has been said above, a preliminary is to establish the premorbid condition. If the patient has been suffering from dementia (Chapter 9), or previously been severely incapacitated with a very poor quality of life, then heroic measures to sustain life are not justified. If the decision to treat is taken, management should aim at maintaining vital functions and preventing complications associated with severe incapacity. Ventilation is ensured by positioning him correctly, and, if necessary, inserting an airway. His swallowing reflex should be tested, and, if this is defective, fluids should be given by a narrow bore nasogastric tube or by intravenous infusion. It is much more difficult to ensure an adequate nutrient intake, and, in the short term, it may be reasonable to ignore this and only review if the dysphagia persists beyond the first 48 hours or so. Regular turning is essential to prevent pressure sores (Chapter 5), and the limbs should be positioned correctly to prevent contractures or subluxation of the shoulder. If the patient is incontinent and severely incapacitated, catheterisation may be necessary to prevent damage to his skin. Faecal stasis and impaction rapidly develop, and should be prevented by appropriate treatment with suppositories and enemas. There is a considerable risk of the patient developing a deep leg vein thrombosis, and low dose heparin should be administered if this is suspected.

Table 8.3   Grades of disability in cerebrovascular disease

Grade I:	No significant disability (able to carry out all usual duties)
Grade II:	Slight disability (unable to carry out previous activities, but able to look after affairs without assistance)
Grade III:	Moderate disability (requiring some help, but able to walk without assistance)
Grade IV:	Moderately severe disability (unable to walk without assistance and unable to attend to own bodily needs without assistance)
Grade V:	Severe disability (bedridden, incontinent and requiring constant nursing care and attention)

Medical Treatment

No medical treatment is currently available for reversing or reducing local tissue damage associated with a stroke. However, a great deal of money and effort is being put into developing appropriate agents and investigating their efficacy. If there is success in this field it will become increasingly important to define the aetiology of strokes, so that sophisticated investigation techniques such as computed tomography, nuclear magnetic resonance imaging, and positron emission tomography are likely to become mandatory.

In the meantime attention must be devoted to preventing recurrence. The antiplatelet agent, aspirin, is of proven efficacy in both transient ischaemic attacks and completed strokes, and should be given in a dose of 75 mg daily. Hypertension should be treated, but in the first two weeks after a stroke, blood pressure is elevated so that treatment should only be started if the pressure remains high beyond this period. Too drastic a change in pressure may, in fact, precipitate a stroke, so that treatment should err on the side of caution. If there is strong circumstantial evidence that the stroke has been due to an embolism, the patient should be given a coumarin anticoagulant, but this ought to be preceded by computed tomography to exclude even the remote possibility of a cerebral haemorrhage.

Surgery has only a limited role to play in the management of stroke patients. There is evidence that this reduces the risk of stroke in patients with carotid artery stenosis of more than 70%. This implies that patients with transient ischaemic attacks and a carotid artery bruit should be referred for vascular ultrasonography. A further condition requiring surgical intervention is subdural haematoma for which drainage is usually effective.

The Rehabilitation Team

Once and indeed even before the clinical condition of the patient has been stabilised, attention should be given to rehabilitation. This aspect of stroke management exemplifies particularly well the points made in Chapter 5 about the importance of close communication and collaboration between all members of the therapeutic team in the care of elderly patients.

The Rehabilitation Therapists

An early objective of the physiotherapist is to improve balance. Until, at the very least, a patient is able to sit in a chair without support, further progress is impossible. She/he then directs attention to improving function in the affected side. This is an important advance over therapy twenty years ago where treatment concentrated on maximising function on the unaffected side, with the result that patients walked with a grossly abnormal gait and often developed flexor deformities in the leg. Preventing spasticity is almost as important as increasing muscle power. This is achieved by ensuring that, at each joint a balance is kept between flexor and extensor power.

While it is particularly important that the patient regains mobility, upper limb function must be remembered and collaboration with the occupational therapist is useful in devising effective but interesting exercises designed to facilitate fine skill movements. Attention to the shoulder joint and diplomatic advice to other staff on positioning the upper limb, with instruction on how to lift the patient, reduces the risk of damage to the joint.

The occupational therapist works in parallel with the physiotherapist training the patient to dress, wash, feed, and toilet himself. This may involve modifications to his clothing such as using adhesive Velcro in the place of buttons or zips, or replacing shoe laces with elastic. Modification to eating and kitchen utensils may be important. Close collaboration between the occupational therapist, physiotherapist and nurse is necessary so that training patterns reinforce rather than counteract each other.

A further important member of the rehabilitation team is the speech therapist. His/her work starts with an initial evaluation of the nature of a communication disorder, distinguishing between such problems as dementia, and a perceptive or motor aphasia. Attention may then be devoted to developing such skills as word finding, reading or writing, or organising exercises in articulation for patients with dysarthria. Even if speech is not restored, the therapist can help a great deal by training patients to communicate by using a picture board or sign language, and by counselling relatives on tackling problems likely to be associated with dysphasia. He/she can also train relatives and volunteers in ways of encouraging and supporting patients to develop and practise their speech and communication skills. In a few instances, patients can be provided with electronic (Canon) communicators on which they can type messages, but these are beyond the capacity of most elderly stroke patients.

The speech therapist can also put her knowledge of the musculature of the mouth and pharynx to good use in retraining patients with swallowing difficulties.

The Nurse

In hospital, the person who spends most time with the patient is the nurse, and she/he has the important task of reinforcing the training being given and organised by his/her colleagues. Examples are that patients should walk rather than be pushed to the lunch table; that they should dress themselves; and that the nurse should spend time talking to patients with speech difficulties. She/he must also organise the patient's day so that self-care activities, rehabilitation and recreation fit together in such a way that his interest has been maintained, his motivation stimulated and undue fatigue avoided. Another important task is to monitor and report back on progress to other members of the team.

If rehabilitation is effectively organised, it can be expected that, of patients surviving the first 3 weeks, one-quarter will become completely independent; half will walk with an aid and require a limited amount of help with self-care, while the remainder will be chairfast and heavily dependent.

Discharge and Follow-up

Prior to discharge, steps must be taken to ensure that the capacities of a patient are sufficient to cope with the environment to which he will be returning. This may involve members of the rehabilitation team going with him to his home to evaluate the situation. Where necessary they may recommend modifications such as fitting rails, building a ramp or moving the bed downstairs, and may order devices such as a raised toilet seat, a commode or a bedside monkey pole.

Even though a patient is reasonably active at the time of discharge from hospital, it is likely that there will be subsequent deterioration. Over the course of a year a large proportion of patients lose their ability and become increasingly dependent. The general practitioner should arrange regular follow-up, so that deterioration can be recognised as quickly as possible and appropriate remedial action taken, either in the form of modified medical treatment, domiciliary physiotherapy or attendance at a geriatric day hospital.

Even if a patient has some degree of mobility, he often imposes a heavy physical and pyschological strain on his family and carers. His lifestyle may be restricted to wandering around the house and watching television, so that he becomes frustrated, irritable, abusive and difficult to live with. Carers must therefore be cared for and relieved of as much as possible. The Chest, Heart and Stroke Association (now the Stroke Association) led the way in developing "stroke clubs", and organising teams of volunteers to provide rehabilitation, support and entertainment for stroke families under the guidance of speech therapists. The Carers National Association has also been active in promoting schemes to provide relief for carers, while the "Crossroads scheme" has provided a valuable sitting service to allow carers to get out of the house.

Stroke Services

The treatment of stroke illness is one of the most demanding and challenging aspects of medical practice. It requires the skilled interaction of a multidisciplinary team, linking with both hospital and the community. In most parts of the country the reality falls far short of the ideal, with patients being admitted in a haphazard manner into one of a number of general medical or geriatric wards where consultants may or may not have a particular interest in the problem, and where it is likely that rehabilitation services are poorly coordinated. There is increasing pressure for each area of the United Kingdom to have a stroke service run by a single coordinator who would be responsible for the initial investigation and management, the subsequent rehabilitation programme, and the post-discharge follow-up of all patients. It is a task for which many geriatricians would be well suited.

PARKINSON'S DISEASE (Cases 1, 8 and 10)

This is a common condition in geriatric medical practice. The patients tend to fall into two groups. Those whose disease is of comparatively recent onset and those who have had the disease for some years, having developed their first symptoms in their 50s or 60s. In both cases, particularly in the latter group, referral to geriatric medicine is often triggered by the patient's increasing dependence on the help of others to remain at home. The incidence of the condition increases with age reaching a peak between 75 and 84 years and affecting about 1% of the population over 65 years, 8% of these requiring institutional care. Though the disease is slightly more common in men than women, more women have Parkinson's disease because they outnumber men in the elderly population.

The clinical manifestations of Parkinson's disease are a combination of tremor, muscle rigidity and generalised poverty of movement (hypokinesia). The tremor is at its worst when the patient is at rest (relaxed), improves when purposeful activity is undertaken but increases with emotional stress or tiredness. It is present in about 70% of cases. The rigidity is particularly disabling, the resistance produced by it being compared with that experienced when bending a lead pipe, but when associated with tremor is jerky and called "cog-wheel". When severe, the imbalance of tone leads to the classical flexed posture, so that the patient is bent forward when walking, with arms held rigidly at the sides, accelerating with small shuffling steps (festination) in a perpetual battle to try and keep up with himself and his centre of gravity. Poverty of movement manifests itself as an expressionless face, motionless arms and slow, deliberate movements. Walking may be difficult to initiate, so that he may get "stuck to the floor". When he finally starts moving he sometimes suddenly freezes. Communication may become difficult, speech losing volume and becoming monotonous, while writing becomes smaller (micrographia) and less legible. Other symptoms include increased sebaceous gland secretion, dehydration, constipation (Chapter 14) and dribbling, due partly to excessive salivation as well as inability to swallow saliva (dysphagia). Thought processes are sometimes slow (bradyphrenia) and the mood flat. A proportion of patients develop a frank dementia, but this usually occurs late in the disease. Depression also is extremely common. At autopsy, loss of neurones can be identified in the substantia nigra and basal nuclei. This is accompanied by a gross reduction of dopamine, an important neurotransmitter.

Most cases are of unknown aetiology, but a substantial minority result from the use of drugs which include butyrophenone and phenothiazine tranquillisers (drug-induced Parkinsonism). This may be due to blocking of striatal dopamine receptors, thereby unmasking a subclinical deficiency of dopamine associated with ageing. A viral aetiology was originally thought likely because of the occurrence of post-encephalitic Parkinsonism. A variant of the disease was associated with an outbreak of encephalitis in 1927, but there is no evidence that current cases of Parkinson's disease have a viral aetiology. Recently, the finding that Parkinsonism in drug addicts was due to the toxic effects of the metabolism of 1-methyl,4-phenyl,1,2,3,6-tetrahydropyridine (MPTP) has suggested that free radicals may play a part in its causation. Other neurological conditions occurring in old age may be associated with Parkinsonian features and have been called the Parkinsonism-plus syndromes. These include multiple cerebral infarcts, senile dementia of the Alzheimer type (SDAT) (Chapter 9) and progressive supranuclear palsy. It can be difficult to differentiate these from Parkinson's disease and the only solution may be to try anti-Parkinsonian drugs. Close surveillance is essential in that such patients who fail to respond to drug treatment are particularly prone to adverse reactions.

The natural history of the disease is a gradual progression over several years to a state of increased dependency and disability. The rate at which this occurs depends on individual variation, the success of drug treatment and the ability of the remedial therapists involved in rehabilitation and re-enablement. At a late stage of the disease a variety of problems including "end-of-dose" unresponsiveness and the "on/off phenomenon" may develop. In the former the duration of action of drugs is shortened so that there are increased episodes of "freezing". In the latter there are swings between rigidity and severe dyskinesia. Both these problems can be alleviated to some extent by increasing the frequency of doses or using agents with a long duration of action. There often also is damage to the autonomic nervous system, which causes excessive salivation, and may also put the patient at risk from postural hypotension (Chapter 10) and hypothermia (Chapter 13). Death usually results from respiratory infection when a state of severe inanition is reached.

Treatment

Treatment has been revolutionised by the use of levodopa. Following absorption, this reaches the central nervous system where it is converted into the neurotransmitter dopamine by the enzyme decarboxylase. The drug increases mobility, reduces rigidity and tremor, and often relieves coincidental depression. Effective blood concentrations without peripheral side effects are achieved by combining levodopa with an inhibitor (benserazide or carbidopa) of peripheral dopa decarboxylase which does not pass the blood–brain barrier. Levodopa does not arrest Parkinson's disease; it merely reduces the patient's symptoms to a level that enables him to lead an independent, active life before declining into a state of severe disability. Fortunately, perhaps, the drug often allows old people to live long enough to die from other diseases before reaching a terminal phase.

The initial dose should be the lowest possible and the interval between doses as long as possible. Depending on the response, the dose and/or frequency should be increased as gradually as possible, small changes being made at intervals of about 2 weeks until an optimum, stable, state of function is achieved. If adverse effects occur, the dose or interval between doses should be reduced and further tentative attempts made to increase it again after a month's stabilisation. Most patients respond favourably, for a period, which may be as long as 5 years or more. If they do not respond the diagnosis should be questioned. Eventually, however, they will experience "end-of-dose" wearing off effects which, though gradual to begin with, will progress to "on/off phenomena". In these the patient experiences phases of freezing in between periods of reasonable function. These can sometimes be overcome by reducing the dose and increasing its frequency.

In some patients, levodopa may produce an acute hallucinatory state, and when this happens there is no alternative but to cease therapy. With long-term therapy most patients experience adverse reactions, especially dyskinesias, when the dose has to be increased to maintain function. These include bizarre movements of their lips and tongue (fly catcher tongue), postural hypotension, psychiatric disorders such as Lilliputian hallucinations and depression.

At the same time as levodopa is started selegiline, a selective monoamine oxidase type B inhibitor, should be introduced. This drug slows the progression of Parkinson's disease. If patients are already taking levodopa the dose should be reduced by a third before starting selegiline at a fixed dose of 10 mg daily.

In the later stages of the disease amantadine may be added with at least some initial benefit. Unfortunately because of tolerance the benefit is ill sustained. Bromocriptine, a dopamine agonist, may improve "end-of-dose", wearing off and "on/off phenomena" of levodopa but the dose has to be low initially and cautiously titrated upwards. A maximum daily dose in elderly patients would be 20 mg. No real advantages are apparent with the newer dopamine agonists—lysuride, lergotrile or pergolide. Similarly the anticholinergic agents' adverse effects preclude their use in elderly patients with Parkinson's disease.

While there is little doubt that drug treatment has revolutionised the management of the patient with Parkinson's disease, the role that the remedial therapist can play in the management of these patients must not be forgotten. Physiotherapy, occupational therapy and speech therapy all play a part in the proper management of the patient. Ideally, all elderly patients should be fully assessed before levodopa therapy is begun, and treatment preceded by a course of appropriate remedial therapy. This assessment is best conducted at the day hospital, where collaboration between doctor and therapists can achieve the greatest degree of mobility and function, while the need for drug therapy is assessed. The simplest of drug regimens can then be implemented and monitored. Inpatient treatment is associated with a high morbidity and mortality from respiratory tract infection: consequently, relatives should be warned of the risks of intermittent "relief" (respite) hospital admissions should these prove necessary in the later stages of the illness.

INVOLUNTARY MOVEMENTS

Tremor

Not all old people with tremor are suffering from Parkinson's disease. Many have an idiopathic senile tremor. In this, the tremor may be fine and rapid, or coarse and slow. It is absent at rest, and increased by movement or emotion. Though a source of inconvenience the condition is relatively innocuous in that it is not associated with akinesia or rigidity, and does not progress to severe incapacity, though it may interfere with finer tasks like doing up buttons. Occasionally the tremor affects the head and neck as well as the hands. Characteristically, the condition is relieved by alcohol. A less addictive remedy is the beta-blocking agent propranolol. However, the majority of patients require no treatment other than reassurance.

Other causes such as hyperthyroidism, beta-2 agonists or sodium valproate also must be considered.

Chorea and Tardive Dyskinesia

Old people occasionally exhibit involuntary rapid jerking movements of their arms and legs. In a less extreme form the head and neck may be involved. These movements may be inappropriate or appear semi-purposeful and be superimposed on voluntary movements. The patient and relatives may be embarrassed. In the absence of focal physical signs or mental impairment they may be labelled as "senile chorea". A more violent "flinging" of the limbs (ballism) is sometimes seen. It may cause falls and may be associated with cerebrovascular disease. When it is unilateral it is known as hemiballismus. Treatment with tetrabenazine may be indicated in some cases but the dose should be increased with caution since confusion, depression and Parkinsonism are all common side effects.

These conditions need to be differentiated from *tardive dyskinesia* which occurs as an adverse reaction to drugs. Slow writhing movements of the tongue, mouth and lips (orofacial dyskinesia) are the commonest form of presentation, but chorea, ballism and purposeless movements of the legs (akathisia) may also occur. In psychotic patients it is often the result of long-term phenothiazine treatment, but its occurrence is not necessarily dose or time related. Stopping phenothiazine may cause remission in some patients. Other drugs including levodopa, oestrogens, butyrophenones and the antiemetic metoclopramide also may be responsible. Tetrabenazine is a useful treatment.

FALLS (Cases 4 and 5)

An old person who suffers from recurrent falls is at risk from a wide range of conditions ranging from fractures of the proximal femur (Chapter 7), through hypothermia (Chapter 13) to head injury with resulting subdural haematoma. He becomes a source of concern to relatives, who often seek institutionalisation, because they are afraid to leave him alone "in case something happens". For these reasons it is essential that the cause of falls is identified and, where possible, steps taken to reduce the risk. It must be recognised, however, that falls are common at all ages and are a risk of "normal living". The points which need special consideration are as follows:

1. *Ageing.* Age-related diseases increase the risk of falling. Poor eyesight, vestibular degeneration, impaired position sense, proximal muscle weakness and degeneration of the cervical apophyseal joints (Chapter 7) are all common concomitants of old age and reasons why balance may be disturbed. If these are complicated by other disease, particularly neurological, or an inappropriate environment the risk is compounded.

2. *Environment.* Study of the individual's home and lifestyle may help to reduce risk. Many falls occur in the home. Steps may be badly worn, bannisters absent or wrongly sited, rooms may have poor natural and artificial light, and cupboards and coin operated meters may be accessible only by climbing a chair or using steps. Other hazards include wobbly furniture, highly polished floors, loose carpets and mats, and trailing flexes. The general practitioner, district nurse or health visitor should be on the look-out for these hazards, and, where appropriate, diplomatically suggest that the situation be altered. In some instances this may involve private or local authority contractors in a considerable amount of reconstruction, and in extreme cases a move to more suitable housing may have to be suggested. However, in some areas "Care and Repair" and "Staying Put" schemes exist that can help the elderly client remain at home.

3. *Vertigo.* Dizziness is a common complaint in the older patient. It is often used to describe a feeling of unsteadiness rather than the rotational sensation of true vertigo. While the former has many causes, the latter is due to vestibular dysfunction. This may be due to loose otoconia in the inner ear (benign positional vertigo), Ménière's disease (a condition due to an excessive amount of endolymphatic fluid), chronic middle ear disease, previous mastoidectomy, ischaemia, acoustic neuroma and drugs, such as aspirin and loop diuretics. An otolaryngological opinion may be needed if ear disease is suspected. In ischaemia the condition may respond to betahistine hydrochloride. Treatment with diuretics or masking aids may be useful in Ménière's disease. Drugs which control dizziness by sedating the central nervous system work well in younger patients, but should be used with extreme caution in the elderly.

They may reduce the sensation of unsteadiness, but by suppressing righting reflexes may increase the risk of falls. Prochlorperazine (Stemetil) is frequently prescribed but does more harm than good in this situation by producing Parkinsonism.

4. *Drop attacks.* This is a disorder that is more common in women. Classically the patient is unable to give a reason for the fall and the terms "cryptogenic" or "idiopathic" are used to describe the condition. Patients often hurt themselves as a result of the fall depending on where and how they have fallen. Having fallen they have difficulty in getting up from the floor for they seem to have lost postural tonus in the legs and trunk. This is restored once they regain the erect posture and their recovery is complete. Falls occur "out of the blue" and if repeated may destroy confidence and compound loneliness. No clear-cut pathology has been identified and some authorities doubt whether this is a true clinical entity, for careful investigation frequently may suggest another possible reason for the fall. Drop attacks may therefore be part of geriatric medical lore.

5. *Epilepsy.* Falls may be associated with loss of consciousness. While this may have a variety of causes, epilepsy is high on the list, and here an eye-witness account from a relative may be useful. It must be recognised, however, that in old age, epilepsy may not present with the classical picture of an aura followed by convulsions. The patient may simply lose consciousness. If it seems likely that the patient has epilepsy, an attempt should be made to distinguish between that due to cerebrovascular disease and that resulting from a benign or malignant tumour. A careful history and examination accompanied by simple investigations such as a chest X-ray may give the answer. If doubt remains more sophisticated tests such as EEG or CT brain scanning should be considered (Chapter 3). Often a therapeutic trial of an anticonvulsant may give a quicker and more effective answer. However, it must be remembered that an accurate diagnosis is just as important in the older patient, particularly if his mobility and quality of life is dependent on being able to drive.

6. *Cardiovascular disease.* A transient loss of consciousness ("blackout"), and a consequent fall, may result from heart block or episodic or continuous arrhythmias, while syncope preceded by dizziness is often the result of postural hypotension (Chapter 10).

Similarly thromboembolism affecting the cerebral arteries may give rise to TIAs (see above) and ischaemia of the mid-brain may result from sudden movements of the neck altering blood flow in the vertebral arteries.

OTHER NEUROLOGICAL CONDITIONS

Most of the other common neurological diseases are also seen in the older patient. These may have been present for a long time and the patient is only referred because severe incapacity means that he requires a high level of care. Some present for the first time in the old patient. Disorders include motor neurone disease, peripheral neuropathies, multiple sclerosis, subacute degeneration of the spinal cord and neurosyphilis. Their management is the same as in younger age groups but their course may be different. Neurosyphilis is very rare now, but positive serological tests are not uncommon in old people with neurological signs (Case 3). While this finding may be of little significance, suggesting a past but not active infection, treatment with a course of penicillin may improve well-being and performance. It should also be remembered that the need and desire for sexual intercourse does not necessarily diminish in old age and consequently sexually transmitted diseases may occur. The neurological manifestations of AIDS should therefore be borne in mind.

Trauma will also affect the nervous system of old people (Chapter 7). A fall may result in a subdural haematoma. This can be difficult to diagnose, particularly if there is no other evidence of injury such as a scalp laceration or a fractured skull.

Pain of neurogenic origin (neuralgia) is not uncommon and may be difficult to treat. The commonest form is post-herpetic neuralgia following an attack of herpes zoster. Early treatment of herpes zoster may be the most effective way of preventing the neuralgia from occurring. Acyclovir 400 mg five times daily for 7 days, supplemented by local application of acyclovir ointment to skin and acyclovir drops to the eye, if this is involved, should be prescribed. If neuralgia occurs treatment is disappointing. Analgesics, such as paracetamol combined with dextropropoxyphen (co-proxamol), may be effective in controlling attacks and there is some evidence that amitriptyline taken regularly at night may reduce the frequency of attacks. Trigeminal neuralgia is less common. It may respond to carbamazepine (Tegretol) but patients with resistant symptoms may need to be referred to special pain clinics.

FURTHER READING

Allen, C.M.C., Harrison, M.J.G. and Wade, D.J. (1989). *The Management of Acute Strokes*. London: Castle House Publications.

Andrews, K. (1991). *Rehabilitation of the Older Adult*. Sevenoaks: Edward Arnold.

Butler, D.S. (1991). *Mobilisation of the Nervous System*. Edinburgh: Churchill Livingstone.

Davies, P.M. (1990). *Right in the Middle*. Berlin: Springer Verlag.

Koller, C. (1987). *Handbook of Parkinson's Disease*. New York: Marcel Dekker.

Mulley, G.P. (1985). *Practical Management of Stroke*. London: Croom Helm.

Pearce, J.M.S. (1992). *Parkinson's Disease and its Management*. Oxford: Oxford University Press.

Tallis, R. (1989). *The Clinical Neurology of Old Age*. Chichester: John Wiley & Sons.

Tideikoaar, R. (1989). *Falling in Old Age: Its Prevention and Treatment*. New York: Springer.

CHAPTER 9 Mental health

INTRODUCTION

Assessment of the mental state of a patient is essential for a complete medical evaluation and to his future management. As has already been indicated, close collaboration between physician and psychiatrist working in the discipline of health care of the elderly is desirable (Chapter 1); psychological changes occur, so that memory is affected and decision making may be impaired (Chapter 2); and mental illness is common (Chapter 6). It should be noted that psychiatric symptoms are a feature in eight out of the ten case histories described. A brief account of some of the changes that occur in the aged brain is needed.

THE BRAIN IN OLD AGE

The human nerve cell has such highly specialised function that it is unable to reproduce itself. This means that the longer a person lives the more likely are disease and degeneration to result in the death of neurones, and thus a reduction in the total number of brain cells. The brains of old people, therefore, may contain many fewer neurones than those of young people. From a functional viewpoint, however, this finding should be interpreted with caution. Accompanying any reduction in the number of brain cells there is a variable reduction in the concentration of substances involved in nerve transmission within the cerebral cortex and the basal ganglia and brain stem. Various structural changes are also found on histological examination of the cerebral cortex. These include oval plaques of degenerative material between neurones (senile plaques) and tangles of dilated microtubules within neurones (neurofibrillary tangles).

Some old people undergo an accelerated loss of nerve cells resulting in atrophy of the cerebral cortex. Histological examination reveals high concentrations of senile plaques and neurofibrillary tangles, the numbers of which bear a direct relationship to the cognitive impairment of the individual. At a biochemical level there is reduction in enzyme activity specifically related to acetylcholine metabolism. The part of the brain most affected by these changes is the hippocampus, a structure intimately associated with memory processing and storage. There is debate as to whether the condition represents an accelerated form of ageing, or if it is a distinct disease entity. The specific changes in acetylcholine metabolism suggest the latter.

Comparison of young and old subjects suggests that, on average, old people have a lower cognitive ability than their younger counterparts. The apparent effect of ageing shown by cross-sectional studies is exaggerated and confounded by secular and other changes. Thus younger people have been better nourished, starting *in utero*, have had less childhood illness and have had more educational opportunities than earlier generations. In addition a seemingly "normal" population of elderly subjects will contain a number of people with latent senile dementia so that the average level of intellectual function for the population will be lowered. Fluid ("short-term") intelligence probably starts its gentle decline in middle age or earlier whereas crystallised intelligence continues to grow throughout age especially in a stimulating environment. Thus it is that older people have difficulty in learning new skills, but have less difficulty in performing tasks dependent on past experience.

MENTAL CONFUSION

The subtle changes in mental function described above are those associated with "normal" ageing and have been called *benign senile forgetfulness*; they are not the reason why some old people are unable to cope with the everyday activities of life. Such change is indicative of disease rather that the ageing process. Old people are often described as being "confused" or "senile"; in either case a definitive diagnosis must be made by making a full assessment of the patient's condition (Chapters 2 and 3), so that his future management can be planned (Chapter 5).

DELIRIUM (Cases 2 and 7)

Delirium is an acute condition which may be defined as a disordered state of mind with incoherent speech and hallucinations. There is often clouding of consciousness so that the doctor may have difficulty in attracting the attention of the patient, and even greater difficulty in sustaining his interest in the interview. Mental function tends to fluctuate so that it may be worse late in the day and immediately after waking. The patient has little control over emotions, and normally subconscious material. Thus, if normally anxious he may present with terror; if depressed may be suicidal; or if suspicious may be paranoid. (Swearing and bad language may be used by the most unexpected people.) People and objects tend to be misidentified, and material normally presenting in dreams often surfaces as hallucinations.

Management

Fundamental to the management of delirium is the identification of the underlying condition responsible (Table 9.1). The doctor's first difficulty is that information from the patient is likely to be unreliable. People who may be able to give relevant information, therefore, must be found and interviewed. These may include relatives, neighbours, the home help, health visitor, district nurse, social worker and general practitioner (if the patient is in hospital). These people are more easily contacted at the patient's home and, if possible, a home visit should be undertaken before admission. It is also in the home that the doctor will be able to pick up useful clues, such as half consumed bottles of alcohol, cupboards full of drugs, or grossly inadequate heating. A home assessment visit, preferably with the general practitioner, may thus be extremely useful.

Management ultimately is dependent on identifying and treating the cause, but while the medical staff are endeavouring to do this the nursing staff can do a great deal to minimise the disruption and distress by a correct approach to the patient. Agitation is reduced if he can see what is going on and is not disturbed by a lot of background noise. He should be nursed in a well-lit, but quiet room (Case 2). Disorientation is lessened if staff identify themselves, explain any procedures they are going to undertake, and frequently give information about time and surroundings. Visual

Table 9.1   Causes of acute confusion (delirium)

Infective	*Electrolyte imbalance*
Bronchopneumonia	Dehydration
Pyelonephritis	Drugs, e.g. diuretics
Local skin lesions	Renal failure
Abscess (septicaemia)	Hypercalcaemia
Bacterial endocarditis	Hyponatraemia
	Endocrine
	Hypothyroidism
Neurological	Diabetes: hypoglycaemia
Drugs with a central	hyperglycaemia
neurological action	Hyperparathyroidism
"Stroke"	
Cerebral tumour	*Nutritional*
Subdural haematoma	"Cachexia"
Epilepsy	B_{12} deficiency
	Thiamine deficiency
	Folate deficiency
Cardiorespiratory	*Miscellaneous*
Myocardial infarction	Anaesthetic agents
Congestive cardiac failure	Trauma (surgical/accidental)
Pulmonary emboli	Tissue anoxia (gangrene)
Respiratory failure	Sudden isolation
Acute haemorrhage	Poisons, e.g. digitalis

hallucinations are more likely to occur in darkness so that at night a small light should be on in the room. Sounds such as running water are liable to misinterpretation so that the patient should be kept well away from such distractions, e.g. bathrooms, sluices, etc. If the patient seems to be living in the past, going through previous unpleasant experiences, it helps if the family can provide information about these so that staff can given reassurance. Patients may recollect their experience during a period of delirium: "it seemed like a bad dream". Recognition of this by the staff and repeated reassurance is most helpful.

The patient may resist attempts at medication or nursing procedures. Painstaking explanation helps to allay his fears, for he may perceive many contacts as being unwarranted attacks on his security and dignity and medicines as being poisons. Finally he may be irritable because of pain or discomfort. Relief of faecal impaction or urinary retention (Chapter 14), or treatment of a pressure sore (Chapter 5) may make him more comfortable, settled and cooperative.

Drug Treatment

Tranquillisers may be required, but must be given in the correct dosage. Too small a dose will merely produce even more clouding of consciousness and *increase* symptoms. Too large a dose may push the patient into coma, increasing the risk of pressure sores and intercurrent chest infection. If tranquillisers have to be used, it is better to give them on a regular than on an "as required" basis. Lower doses are required to prevent the manifestations of delirium than to control these once they have established themselves. Oral preparations include thioridazine tablets or syrup, haloperidol drops, and chlorpromazine. Intramuscular injections may be necessary and, here, chlorpromazine, promazine or haloperidol may be used. Rarely, in extreme cases prolonged sedation is required. This can be achieved with an intravenous infusion of chlormethiazole, but the rate has to be controlled by a pump, and nursing staff have to keep a constant watch on the level of consciousness.

If the individual is restless at night a hypnotic should be given, but in these cases the dose should be adequate to produce a sound sleep. Otherwise the patient may be left in a limbo of nightmares and hallucinations. The duration of action should be short so that a state of drowsiness does not persist throughout the following day. Chlormethiazole tablets or capsules fulfil these criteria, as do short acting benzodiazepines such as temazepam. Barbiturates and long acting benzodiazepines such as nitrazepam should be avoided in these situations.

DEMENTIA (Case 4)

The simplest definition of dementia is that it is a syndrome of global mental disturbance in an alert patient. It has to be distinguished from the minor brain changes associated with ageing already described, other mental illness, particularly depression, or conditions such as subnormality which may have been lifelong.

Prevalence

It has been said that severe mental decay, on account of the state of extreme helplessness it produces in its later stages, constitutes the largest single problem in the field of care of the elderly. After the age of 65 years it shows an exponential rise in both men and women from less than 5% in those aged 65 to 69 years, to over 20% in those over 80 years (Figure 9.1). Though the prevalence is similar for a given age in the two sexes, at the present time there are many more women than men affected, since in this older age group women outnumber men by three to one (Chapter 1).

Aetiology

While there are many possible causes of dementia in old age, 85% of a consecutive series of autopsies of patients, average age 77 years, with a clinical diagnosis of dementia either had senile dementia or multi-infarct dementia or a mixture of the two conditions, 8% had no discernable lesion while the remaining 7% had other disorders. Those with "senile dementia" had changes similar

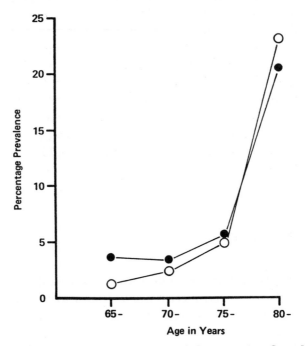

Figure 9.1 Prevalence of chronic brain failure in men ● and women ○

to those seen in Alzheimer's disease. The histological changes of classical Alzheimer's disease seen in younger subjects in their late 50s and early 60s tend to be more severe than those that occur in older patients. Cell loss in the subcortical nuclei is also greater. Structural changes are more marked than those due to ageing, senile plaques occurring in greater numbers in the cerebral cortex, as do neurofibrillary tangles (NT) in both cortex and hippocampus. Similarly, the severity of biochemical changes correlates with the structural changes. It also follows a more malignant clinical course, with associated neurological changes such as dysphasia, apraxia and extrapyramidal signs being more common, and with a striking reduction in life expectancy. For this reason the more benign dementia in old people is described as being "senile dementia of the Alzheimer type" (SDAT).

In about a quarter of elderly patients with dementia there is a vascular cause with the brain containing multiple cerebral infarcts, resulting from high blood pressure, atheroma and thromboembolic episodes, but cognitive impairment does not become apparent usually until more than 100 ml of brain tissue has been lost. This intellectual impairment due to a patchy destruction of brain tissue is described as multi-infarct dementia (MID). It occurs more frequently in men, tends to affect a slightly younger age group than SDAT, and produces stepwise clinical deterioration. It is also associated more frequently with neurological abnormalities, patchy cognitive impairment and emotional lability. Parkinsonian features particularly the short stepping gait may be present (Chapter 8). Brain scans, CT or MRI (Chapter 3) show ventricular enlargement, widened sulci, cerebral infarcts and white matter changes.

Finally the remaining 15% of patients with dementia either have no histological abnormality or suffer from one of the wide range of disorders listed in Table 9.2. Though small this group is important since it may include conditions that can be prevented, treated or even reversed. It also includes some progressive dementias without Alzheimer changes, including diffuse Lewy body disease and the leucoencephalopathies. In the former condition memory loss is an early feature and psychotic symptoms become prominent as the disease progresses, particularly hallucinations, depression and aggressive behaviour.

Natural History

One of the earliest features of SDAT is poor memory for recent events. This often is accompanied by disabilities in abstract thinking, judgement and self-criticism. In the early stages these changes may be indistinguishable from variants of normality, so that it is often relatives rather than professionals who first identify the alteration in cognitive function and personality.

As the condition progresses forgetfulness becomes more serious so that, instead of merely forgetting names, the patient may forget to switch off a cooker, or go out into the street inappropriately dressed. At this stage variations in personality become accentuated so that a forthright person may become rude, a forceful individual aggressive and a timid patient tearful and agitated. In some instances, a strong personality may serve to disguise underlying impairment. Hence, a gregarious old lady will continue to chat cheerfully to her friends, and it may be some time before they realise that she is talking nonsense. If unable to give the right answer she obligingly makes one up (confabulates) and presents a seemingly normal social facade. An arthritic old lady in a long-stay ward may say that she has been out shopping all morning, and that she has come home to cook her mother's lunch. In other cases, supported direction from a spouse may mask the condition which only becomes apparent when something happens to the able partner.

At a later stage of the disease there are serious changes in behaviour. The patient dresses untidily, eats sloppily, and gives up any attempt to cook or do housework. He may urinate or defaecate in the wrong places or simply become incontinent of urine and faeces. Wandering is often a problem, in that the patient may visit rela-

Table 9.2   Causes of dementia

Alzheimer's disease	Hypothyroidism
Multiple cerebral infarcts	Chronic alcoholism
Jakob–Creutzfeldt disease	Chronic dialysis
Pick's disease	Huntington's chorea
Neurosyphilis	Parkinson's disease
Leucoencephalopathies	Progressive supranuclear palsy
Hydrocephalus	Wernicke's encephalopathy
Cerebral tumour	Post-traumatic (boxers)
Diffuse Lewy body disease	B_{12} deficiency
Meningioma	Subdural haematoma

tives or go shopping in the middle of the night, and then forget why he has come out or where he lives.

In the final stages, extensive cerebral damage results in the patient developing muscle weakness, spasticity, ataxia, and flexion contractures. He lies permanently curled up in bed, his only response to stimuli being to grasp or suck things. Mercifully the patient then usually develops bronchopneumonia and dies.

There is a considerable variation in the rate at which patients with SDAT deteriorate. In some old people the progress is very slow, forgetfulness being the main feature. Initially there may be doubt as to whether this is a normal variant of ageing or an early stage of dementia. The doctor should be aware of this, identify the patient as being "at risk", keep him under review, and be cautious with the prognosis.

Diagnosis

A diagnosis of dementia can usually be made by taking a careful history from relatives and, sometimes, neighbours. Figure 9.2 illustrates the steps that should be taken in order to reach the diagnosis. Depression and lifelong mental handicap (retardation) must be recognised for the former can be treated and the latter managed. In assessing prognosis and planning support it is useful to try and quantify the severity of the impairment. Aspects which should be covered include orientation in time, place and people, memory for recent and distant events, and numeracy. This can be done by using a simple, short questionnaire. A considerable amount of research has been undertaken in recent years to find which of the many questionnaires in use is likely to be the most useful. Those most commonly used are the information/orientation (IO) sub-test of the Clifton Assessment Procedure for the Elderly (CAPE), the Mini-Mental State Examination (MMSE) and the Abbreviated Mental Test (AMT) (Table 9.3), which is probably the easiest to use. All vary in their sensitivity, specificity and positive predictive value, depending on the "cut off point" used. Some other conditions such as mental handicap, depression, deafness and dysphasia may produce low scores in all these tests and must be recognised. Finally, patients admitted to hospital tend to be flustered and may score badly while those with acute illness may be confused (delirium) (Case 7). Tests, therefore, should be used to supplement rather than replace overall clinical judgement in diagnosing dementia, as well as being used to monitor the progress of the condition.

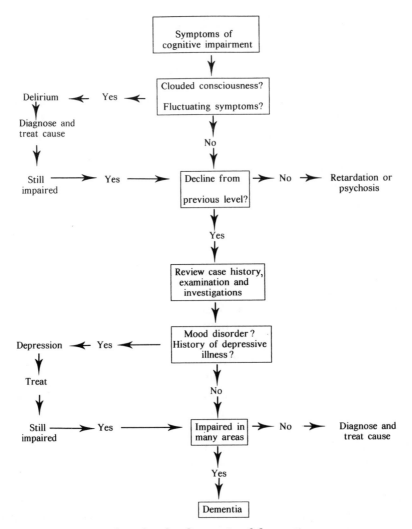

Figure 9.2   Steps taken for the diagnosis of dementia

Another important dimension of dementia is behaviour. In assessing this, performance in a spectrum of tasks is scored in grades from 1–5. Tasks include dressing, feeding, toileting, communication and activity disturbance. The system is useful in providing both a pattern and overall score for behavioural abnormality.

Table 9.3   The Abbreviated Mental Test

1. Age
2. Time
3. Address recall, e.g. 42 West Street
4. Year
5. Place
6. Recognition of two persons
7. Date of birth
8. Year of World War I
9. Name of monarch
10. Count 20–1

Note: Cut off point 7/8 gives highest sensitivity and specificity.

Management

It has been said that in the presence of brain damage, man may use any strategy to achieve his end. Indeed the creation of a strategy is the most important part of management. Having made sure that the diagnosis is correct and that no remediable condition has been missed, a long-term management plan has to be made.

Drug treatment

In SDAT and MID there are no drugs which produce a significant improvement in mental function. Identification of an agent that will do this awaits the outcome of future clinical trials with all their inherent problems in the elderly. This does not mean that drugs have no place in the management of dementia. Phenothiazines may be useful if the patient is agitated or inclined to wander. Optimum and regular dosage is critical, since undersedation leads to disinhibition and increased restlessness, while oversedation will lead to sleepiness, falls and immobility. If a careful history is taken or the patient closely observed, it often is possible to chose optimal times for administration of an agent. A hypnotic such as chlormethiazole or temazepam may be useful in controlling nocturnal restlessness. Their relatively short duration of action means that excessive drowsiness the following morning should not be a problem. Since depression often accompanies dementia, when insight is preserved, judicious use of antidepressants may be very helpful in relieving suffering.

Social support

Over 80% of demented patients live in their own homes, and places in residential homes, nursing homes and mental hospitals are over-subscribed. As stated earlier (Chapter 4), it is the policy of most health and social services agencies to maintain people at home for as long as possible. This places a considerable burden on the carer. Support services must be directed not only toward the patient but also toward the carer. If we are to expect a carer to carry the burden imposed by the demented individual then the management plan must be agreed between the carer and those whose duty it is to provide the support. Since in the future (after April 1993), this will become the responsibility of the social services department of the local authority, clear guidelines will have to be written as to "who does what", so that the monitoring and audit of services can be undertaken. Help will consist of giving advice to ensure the carer is in receipt of the statutory allowances, grants and services available, so that he is in a position to help himself as much as possible. The primary medical care team should undertake to moni-tor, with the community psychiatric nurse and the psychogeriatric team, the clinical state of the patient and the stress placed upon the carer. Support services, such as the home help, day centre and day hospital relief, continence advisory and laundry service, sitting services and respite care, all need to be available and their use planned, as far as is possible for that individual patient. Counselling should also be available, formally and informally, for carers because of the very considerable emotional stress to which they may be subjected. Care managers may have an important role in commissioning and monitoring such services (Chapter 4).

Carers will be more likely to keep the patient at home and share care if they know that when a crisis arises they will get relief immediately. Unless this can be guaranteed some carers may be unwilling to take on the burden of responsibility. Support by the local voluntary Alzheimer Disease Society can be invaluable.

Unfortunately, there is a rising proportion of old people with mental impairment who do not have family support. Sheltered housing, with support from social services, may help to contain the situation. Particular attention may need to be given to prob-lems, such as wandering or leaving gas taps on, which may cause disturbance or create danger for others. These can be tackled if they are recognised and clearly defined. For example, ensuring a safe enclosed area, where people can wander, yet remain within the confines of the housing complex or fitting fail-safe gas taps. Even with these, however, long-term institutionalisation is usually necessary at an earlier stage than in patients with families.

Long-term Care

In spite of the attempt to keep a patient in his own home, the time may come when institutional care is required. If possible this should be preplanned. Ideally, placement in residential accommodation should be attempted and the establishment of homes for the elderly mentally infirm (EMI) may be justified. These homes can cater for people with mild to moderate dementia who may or may not have considerable physical disability. They require special architectural design and colour schemes and if supported either by hospital specialists or interested general practitioners, a good environment can be engendered. This in turn, has a favourable effect on the symptoms of the disease as well as staff morale and recruitment. In such homes, classical custodial care regimes can be abandoned and attempts made to encourage residents to maintain as independent a role for the activities of daily living as is compatible with their condition. The more this is developed the more surprising it is how individuals do and can respond to the positive approach. This has obvious benefits for both residents and staff.

The satisfactory placement of patients with dementia in a home or hospital, whether this be private, voluntary or statutory, depends not only on the degree of their behavioural disturbance and physical disabilities, but also on the tolerance and training of the caring staff. Further, whether residents should be grouped together in a wing or randomly placed throughout the home is a question which will depend on design and local circumstances. A clear policy, however, must be agreed and followed so that an elderly subject with dementia is placed in an environment appropriate to his needs. The provision of an adequate psychogeriatric service which achieves liaison between the hospital and the community helps to avoid these placement conflicts, with benefit to the patient and a greater efficiency in the use of expensive resources.

The management of severe dementia should follow similar principles, whether the individual is in hospital or nursing home. To this end patients should be constantly encouraged to feed themselves at the table, and mobility, even with its attendant risks, should be encouraged. The physical environment should either be adapted or designed with these in mind. A large well-lit and well-decorated day room is mandatory. Vivid door colourings can be used to identify toilet areas; similarly, bed coverings should be coloured to enable patients to find their own beds. The whole atmosphere of the patient's day should be focused towards activity. Corridors should be "staggered" at a central point to break up the appearance of length, without obscuring observation, to allow for wandering. Garden areas should have paved paths, be secure and connect with the internal circulation space.

For adequate care and stimulation a high staff : patient ratio is required, though not all staff need to be professionals. Voluntary workers or relatives should be encouraged to participate in the patient's activities and to suggest activities of their own. Relatives should be consulted to determine the various premorbid preferences of the patients. Not all patients enjoy playing bingo, watching television or joining in sing-songs, and individual preferences should be catered for. In order to attempt to orientate the patients to the passage of time, frequent trips outside the hospital or home will allow some to appreciate the changing seasons; raised gardens that patients can work themselves are useful, and may uncover hidden ability. Other activities include painting, playing the piano or other musical instrument, or making things like soft toys. These activities and many others require materials with which some patients will be able to interact. Not all these activities need highly skilled professional staff. Though a nucleus of such staff is essential, time and positive attitudes are the most valuable attributes. For example, a very demented old lady, who had been a good pianist, would when seated at the paino play the first eight bars of a piece of music. If someone sat beside her and prompted her, encouraging her to play on, she would do so. With continuing constant encouragement and persuasion she would eventually play the whole piece, something she clearly enjoyed doing. Many units for the elderly severely mentally infirm (ESMI), find school children and students are often willing to help with this sort of activity, and patients themselves seem to relate well to the younger age groups.

OTHER MENTAL ILLNESS

Depression (Cases 1, 3, 6, 8 and 9)

This topic has already been discussed in Chapter 6. It is mentioned again here to emphasise its high prevalence and the overlap of symptoms with those of dementia. Depression, often severe, may present as dementia (pseudodementia). It responds to treatment with antidepressants but sometimes may require unipolar electro-convulsant therapy (ECT). Patients may require to continue anti-depressants for long periods to prevent relapse. Tricyclic and tetra-cyclic agents and the newer 5-HT uptake inhibitors are the most effective drugs. Other antidepressants, such as lithium, tryptophan and monoamine oxidase inhibitors, should not be used in the eld-erly unless prescribed by a psychiatrist. Many elderly patients with disability suffer from an associated depressive illness which responds gratifyingly to antidepressants.

Neurosis

Neurosis which has occurred at a younger age may persist into old age or occur for the first time. It may give rise to isolation and subnutrition. Treatment is similar to the younger patient, but particular care should be taken if benzodiazepine tranquillisers are prescribed since these often cause neuropsychiatric side effects and habituation.

Paraphrenia

This condition is often associated with deafness and impaired vision in the older patient. He may suffer from visual and auditory hallucinations. He will complain of "heads popping out of walls" or of voices coming from "upstairs" or "next door", sometimes accusing him of immoral or dishonest behaviour, which may make him withdraw from society and because a recluse. The condition responds to phenothiazines which, if they do not make the heads disappear or voices go away, alter their threat or content so that the "nasty" sayings become "nice".

FURTHER READINGS

Arie, T. (ed.) (1992). *Recent Advances in Psychogeriatrics—2*. Edin-burgh: Churchill Livingstone.
Jacoby, R. and Oppenheim, C. (1991). *Psychiatry in the Elderly*. Oxford: Oxford University Press.

Jacques, A. (1988). *Understanding Dementia*. Edinburgh: Churchill Livingstone.

Lindsay, J. MacDonald, A. and Starke, I. (1990). *Delirium in the Elderly*. Oxford: Oxford University Press.

Marshall, M. (1990). *Working with Dementia—Guidelines for Professionals*. Birmingham: Venture Press.

Stuart-Hamilton, I. (1991). *The Psychology of Ageing*. London: Jessica Kingsley.

CHAPTER 10 The cardiovascular system

AGEING AND AGE-RELATED CHANGES

It is very difficult to disentangle the effects of biological ageing of the cardiovascular system from the effects of age-related atherosclerosis. It is the interaction of the two processes which leads to the very high prevalence of cardiovascular problems in elderly people of developed nations. As other global areas adopt Western lifestyles, it is likely that cardiovascular disease, as yet relatively infrequent in their ageing populations, will become more of a problem in the very near future (Chapter 1). Using the criteria of ageing described in Chapter 1 and studying so-called primitive human populations not (as yet) assaulted by atherosclerosis, some ageing changes can be clearly differentiated from age-related diseases. These data are complemented by animal work which unfortunately is often confused by interspecies differences.

Morphological Changes

There is almost a linear increase in deposition of fat, fibrous tissue, lipofuscin and amyloid in both ventricles of the heart, particularly the left. It is probable that the accumulation of lipofuscin, a waste product of cellular metabolism, has no functional significance. The other changes, however, do decrease the contractility of individual muscle fibres and decrease compliance (increase stiffness). The left ventricle is affected more than the right ventricle because of its higher work load, due to the higher systemic vascular pressures. In extreme old age, i.e. above 95 years of age, the accumulation of amyloid may lead to chronic heart failure. The heart valves also undergo ageing changes though some of these are purely the result of repetitive mechanical trauma. In the aortic valve stiffness associated with the accumulation of collagen may progress to calcification. This increases the pressure gradient across the valve with a resultant systolic murmur. This is often dismissed as benign due to "aortic sclerosis". Such a diagnosis leads to complacency. Good echocardiographic (Chapter 3) evidence exists that many of these patients have stenosis, which may be improved by operation (see later). Patients with aortic systolic murmurs, therefore, require regular follow-up.

The mitral valve tends to dilate gradually with increasing age though it is unlikely to become incompetent without additional factors (infection, infarction). The conducting system of the heart, however, is affected by age changes, particularly those affecting collagen and the deposition of fibrous tissue. This may cause significant conduction disturbances, such as bradyarrhythmias and heart block, in the absence of significant atherosclerosis.

Major peripheral arteries also are subject to the ageing process. Fibrous tissue accumulates making them less compliant and more dilated. This particularly applies to the aorta. Unfolding of the aortic arch may be seen on routine chest radiography and must not be confused with aneurysmal dilatation. The reduction in elasticity increases the likelihood of intimal tears and also leads to an increased systolic blood pressure and a wider pulse pressure.

Physiological Changes   (Table 10.1)

The morphological changes in the left ventricle, which increase its stiffness, impair diastolic function. The ability to accelerate the heart rate during stress (exercise, fever, shock etc.) is attenuated with increasing age. The maximum heart rate for an individual can best be estimated by the formula—220 minus his age in years. The combination of a reduction in stroke volume and heart rate leads to a reduction in cardiac output (litres per minute). It is, however, becoming apparent from well-conducted studies in humans, that the previous estimates for reduction in cardiac output with increasing age were exaggerated. This was due, mainly, to the confounding effects of both latent and apparent disease.

The reduction in stroke volume is due to the age-related morphological changes. Thus, the Frank–Starling curve of a healthy elderly patient is flatter and shifted to the right compared with a younger individual. This limits the reserve capacity of the heart to respond to increased demands for a cardiac output. However, other

Table 10.1   Functional decreases due
to ageing

Maximal heart rate
Systolic function (minor)
Diastolic function (major)
Stroke volume
Cardiac output
Oxygen consumption
    (related to lean body mass)

changes in the aged individual (reduction in lean body mass and basal metabolic rate) lead to a reduction in the demands for a cardiac output. Consequently, with normal ageing, a crude balance between demand and supply for cardiac output is maintained. Hence, the ageing changes that affect the cardiovascular system should not lead to significant symptoms even in patients over the age of 85 years. Therefore, the old person who becomes breathless walking on the flat is likely to be in decompensated chronic cardiac failure or suffering from a respiratory disorder such as chronic bronchitis, emphysema or bronchial asthma (Chapter 11).

ATHEROSCLEROTIC DISEASE IN THE ELDERLY
(Case 3)

The precise aetiology of this disease is unknown but it is obvious that multiple genetic and environmental factors are involved (Table 10.2). The disease starts early in life, the environment *in utero* and in the first year of life perhaps playing a part in setting appropriate conditions for its development, there usually being a long latent period (30+ years) before cardiovascular symptoms are manifested. There is evidence that by changing lifestyle the prevalence and progression of atherosclerosis can be reduced. In particular, the reduction in smoking, especially cigarettes, in populations has resulted in cardiovascular benefit. The precise contribution made by the modification of other factors in Table 10.2 is less certain.

Atherosclerosis may involve the coronary arteries leading to a reduction in the supply of oxygen and other metabolic nutrients to working cardiac muscle. Consequences include angina pectoris, myocardial infarction and/or chronic cardiac failure. The first sign of coronary artery disease in elderly people may be a cardiac

Table 10.2   Factors affecting atherosclerosis

Smoking	Obesity
Hypertension	High saturated fat diet
Lack of exercise	Familial hyperlipidaemia
Diabetes mellitus	Hypothyroidism
Endothelial trauma	High levels of free radicals

arrhythmia. This may be persistent, paroxysmal or transient. The elevation of blood pressure with increasing age may accelerate the development of atherosclerotic lesions, which in turn lead to a further increase in blood pressure producing a vicious circle. Manifestation of atherosclerotic lesions in peripheral arteries include symptoms and signs of vascular insufficiency and even frank gangrene. The effects of lesions in the cerebral arteries are described in Chapter 8.

CORONARY ARTERY DISEASE (Case 7)

Prevention

At present our inability to reverse atherosclerosis requires that we seek ways of preventing or slowing the progression of the disease. In elderly patients this may seem like "closing the stable door after the horse has bolted". Preventative measures should be aimed at young populations—reducing smoking, lowering lipids by diet or drugs, promoting exercise, reducing obesity. Even in patients over the age of 65 years, and particularly those at risk, these measures are effective in reducing the morbidity and mortality (Table 10.2). The most effective are to avoid or stop smoking, and to control both diastolic and systolic hypertension. Although there is less firm evidence on the efficacy of physical exercise, the reduction of obesity, an increased intake of ascorbic acid or vitamin E, or the reduction of hypercholesterolaemia by dietary measures, it seems prudent to advise old people to take a moderate amount of exercise (Chapter 6), to control their weight, to avoid high cholesterol foods and to take plenty of fruit and vegetables. Also hypothyroidism and non-insulin dependent diabetes mellitus (Chapter 13) should be identified and controlled, though even tight treatment of the latter does not benefit macrovascular atherosclerosis.

ANGINA

Atherosclerotic lesions in the coronary vessels impair blood supply to the working myocardium. When the work of the heart increases during exercise, the coronary arteries may deliver insufficient oxygenated blood producing cardiac anoxia. This generates the sensation of precordial pain felt often by the patient as a tight constricting band round the chest. It may radiate up into the throat or down the left or both arms. The characteristic of anginal pain is that it is relieved promptly by rest and the exercise required to produce the symptoms is predictable. It is rarely necessary to study exercise ECGs to make the diagnosis. Approximately 10% of individuals over the age of 80 years suffer from angina and there is no male preponderance, such as occurs in younger age groups. Occasionally elderly patients may suffer from angina decubitus, i.e. anginal pain brought on by lying flat. This needs to be distinguished from orthopnoea or oesophageal reflux (Chapter 12). Rarely patients may suffer angina after eating a meal (postprandial).

Treatment of angina in the elderly consists of glycerol trinitrate in the form of a spray as this reduces the total dose and hence the adverse effects (headache, flushing, faintness). Long acting nitrates, such as isosorbide mononitrate, may be useful in some patients. Occasionally it is necessary to off-load the work of the heart by using a calcium antagonist (nifedipine, diltiazem) or a beta-blocker (propranolol, oxprenolol). But both groups of drugs can produce myocardial depression and cardiac failure in elderly patients. They may worsen bradyarrhythmias and peripheral vascular disease, while even the cardioselective beta-1-adrenoceptor blocking drugs (atenolol, metoprolol) can increase airways resistance in susceptible individuals (see paragraph on asthma in "Obstructive syndromes", Chapter 11).

Often in elderly patients, anginal symptoms can be managed by altering the environment. The provision of a shopping assistant, a home help or a stair lift may reduce the work on the heart. The cardiac surgeon and the cardiologist may be able to make valuable contributions to treatment and old people, whose health is good otherwise, should not be deprived of coronary artery bypass grafting or percutaneous transluminal coronary angioplasty. The decision should be based on the quality of the patient's life and his physiological state. Results are usually excellent.

MYOCARDIAL INFARCTION (Case 7)

Presentation

Approximately 30% of elderly patients with myocardial infarction present with the classical features of an acute onset with crushing retrosternal chest pain often radiating up into the jaw/teeth and down the left arm. It is associated with faintness or frank syncope and the pain usually lasts more than one hour. These symptoms are invariably recognised by both patient and his relatives as being those of a "coronary thrombosis". A further 30% of patients present atypically and without any chest pain. Such patients may become suddenly breathless, complain of generalised weakness (take to their bed) or develop recurrent falls and present with trauma. Alternatively the patient may become suddenly disorientated and confused. In these situations the doctor requires a high degree of clinical acumen, and should perform an ECG and, if necessary, take blood for cardiac enzyme estimation to confirm the diagnosis. The only clue to the diagnosis is the speed of onset of symptoms. The final third of patients have a silent myocardial infarction. They have no significant symptoms and do not present to medical services. They are only discovered by accident, when a routine electrocardiograph shows an abnormal pattern compatible with old myocardial infarction or change from a previously normal tracing. It used to be thought that silent myocardial infarction only occurred in the very old. Increasingly, however, it is apparent that silent infarcts occur in younger people. There is no clear explanation why infarction in these individuals is pain-free. The malign comment that elderly patients do not feel pain is not borne out by observation. If older individuals have been affected by coronary artery disease for longer they may have developed a better collateral circulation thus minimising any myocardial damage. Additionally, it may be that autonomic changes decrease sensitivity.

Management

No longer can elderly patients with acute myocardial infarction be routinely treated at home and denied the benefits of high technology medicine. Because the mortality and morbidity of acute myocardial infarction are higher in elderly patients, the benefits of active intervention are also proportionally higher. In the few instances where, prior to the infarction, an elderly patient has been mentally and/or physically severely disabled, he may be kept in homely surroundings within the community and treated conservatively with analgesics. In all other cases it is quite clear that the elderly benefit *more* from intensive treatment than do younger patients. Perhaps this is a situation where reverse ageism applies! Patients should be admitted promptly to the nearest coronary care unit and treated with thrombolytic therapy (streptokinase) and aspirin. Early treatment reduces both immediate and late mortality and, most importantly, reduces morbidity by improving left ventricular function. Analgesia needs to be given and the dose titrated against the response in pain-relief. Very high doses of narcotic analgesics are required in some elderly individuals and those with chronic respiratory disease may be more sensitive to the respiratory depressant effect of narcotics so that this must be monitored. Other complications of acute myocardial infarction such as arrhythmias, cardiac failure and shock should be treated as necessary.

For many an elderly patient admission to a coronary care unit is his first experience of hospital. He will be anxious and probably intimidated by the technology. He must be apprised of his illness, told in clear, understandable and optimistic terms, what is happening, and reassured. The objective is to remobilise him as soon as his general condition permits, usually within 24 hours. Rapid rehabilitation prevents the problems of dependency and immobility and speeds discharge. Obviously this has considerable psychological benefits. Long-term therapy, with a low dose of aspirin (75 mg daily) is beneficial but beta-blockers are best avoided because of the risk of cardiac failure. Smokers, particularly cigarette smokers, should be advised to stop since this has been shown to be beneficial even in extreme old age. Other preventive measures are less likely to be effective, though patients should be encouraged to review their previous way of life and take into consideration those risk factors already discussed above.

CARDIAC FAILURE (Cases 2, 5, 7 and 10)

There are no differences in management of acute onset cardiac failure in elderly patients compared with younger ones. However, the management (diagnosis and treatment) of chronic cardiac failure in old age is different.

Diagnosis

It must be remembered that cardiac failure is not in itself a primary diagnosis and some causes of chronic cardiac failure which commonly present in old age are given in Table 10.3. A detailed search for these causes which may be acting independently or contributing to cardiac failure is well worthwhile as direct treatment has obvious benefits for elderly patients. It should not be assumed that all cases of chronic cardiac failure in old age are due to irreversible coronary artery disease.

The diagnosis is straightforward when the patient presents with congestive symptoms related to an increased left ventricular end diastolic pressure, such as increasing dyspnoea of effort, orthopnoea and paroxysmal nocturnal dyspnoea, and, on examination, is found to have a raised jugular venous pressure, cardiomegaly, hepatomegaly, dependent oedema, and basal crepitations. However, because of the altered Frank–Starling relationship, described earlier, an elderly patient may present more with the symptoms of a low cardiac output. Thus he may complain of non-specific weakness, tiredness, lethargy, fatigability and "take to his bed". On occasions he may present with rapidly increasing confusion, or with bronchopneumonia, a complication of chronic cardiac failure which neither the patient nor his doctor has recognised. Alternatively, chronic cardiac failure may be over-diagnosed. There are

Table 10.3   Aetiology of chronic cardiac failure

Coronary artery disease
Hypertension
Valvular disease
Drugs, e.g. beta-blockers
                 calcium channel antagonists
Arrhythmias
Chronic obstructive airways disease
Pulmonary hypertension (emboli)
Cardiomyopathies
High output
    anaemia
    thiamine deficiency
    thyrotoxicosis
    AV fistula
    nephritis
    Paget's disease of bone
Primary amyloid

many causes of pitting oedema of the lower limbs (Table 10.4) and it cannot be overemphasised that immobility is a potent cause. The treatment is remobilisation and not diuretics. Not all basal creptitations heard at the lung bases are due to left ventricular failure. If they disappear on coughing they are physiological (Chapter 11). Similarly raised jugular venous pressure may be the consequence of raised intrathoracic pressure due to chronic bronchitis, and hepatomegaly in old age has many causes. Chronic cardiac failure and its degree is best ascertained by a detailed history and functional (exercise) assessment combined with a good posteroanterior (PA) chest X-ray which will show cardiomegaly, upper lobe blood flow diversion and basal congestion. Echocardiography (Chapter 3) may also be helpful in elucidating the cause.

Treatment

The mainstay of treatment of chronic cardiac failure in old age is a diuretic agent. Because of the age-related decrement in renal function (Chapter 13) associated with a further decrease in the glomerular filtration rate due to reduced cardiac output, thiazide agents are relatively ineffective. However, high doses of potent loop agents are not usually required. Even in acute pulmonary oedema diuresis is established and pulmonary pressures lowered with small intravenous doses. This applies also to chronic cardiac failure. A torrential diuresis does not particularly benefit the cardiovascular system, may ruin a perfectly good carpet and totally destroy the patient's morale. Equally, patients will not continue to comply for long with drugs that render them tethered to the toilet or, at worst, incontinent. Small doses, e.g. bumetanide 0.5 mg or frusemide 20 mg, can be given either once or twice daily. Also the patient must be told that he can take the drug at any time to suit his daily programme. So often he is told that he *must* take his tablet first thing in the morning, with the result that he is frightened to leave

Table 10.4 Causes of lower limb oedema in the elderly

Immobility	Venous obstruction
Cardiac failure	Hepatic cirrhosis
Nephrotic syndrome	Incompetent venous valves
Hypoalbuminaemia	Pelvic mass (tumour, faeces)
Leg vein surgery	

the house for the next 6 hours. If there are outside events he wishes to attend during this time there is no reason why he should not take the drug at a more convenient time. The patient will soon learn the duration of the drug's effect and can take the dose to accord with the structure of his day. This is far better than repeated omission of doses.

For patients who do not respond to the initial low dose of loop agent, increasing doses should be tried. Simultaneously a review of the diagnosis and factors contributing to the cardiac failure should be undertaken (Table 10.3). Compliance should also be checked. If the chronic cardiac failure is truly resistant to treatment then diuresis can often be induced by adding in the diuretic metolazone on a short-term basis. This can cause severe electrolyte depletion which must be monitored. Alternatively, an angiotensin-converting enzyme (ACE) inhibitor can be added but, because of the danger of sudden hypotension, the diuretic agent should be withdrawn or, at least, its dosage halved for 24 hours before starting the ACE inhibitor. Blood pressure should be monitored for up to 6 hours before starting an ACE inhibitor in any patient who is on high dose diuretic therapy. Indeed, it is useful to start off with a test dose of 6.25 mg of captopril. Other drugs are of limited use in the treatment of chronic cardiac failure in old people. The adverse effects of digoxin (Case 7) outweigh any potential benefits in those patients who are in sinus rhythm. It should be reserved for the treatment of fast atrial fibrillation (see below). The metabolic adverse effects of diuretics (Table 10.5) have been exaggerated in the past, particularly hypokalaemia, which frequently predates the use of diuretics. If an elderly patient taking diuretics does become significantly hypokalaemic (serum potassium less than 3.0 mmol/l) then an alternative cause should be sought. In particular, gastro-intestinal loss (laxative abuse or diarrhoea) should be considered.

Table 10.5   Metabolic effects of diuretic agents*

Hyperkalaemia (+ sparing agent)
Hyponatraemia
Uraemia
Hypokalaemia
Hyperglycaemia
Hypercalciuria
Hyperuricaemia

*NB: More likely with thiazide than loop agents.

The adverse effects profile of so-called potassium sparing agents, including renal impairment, hyperkalaemia and hyponatraemia, suggests that these drugs should not be used.

CARDIAC ARRHYTHMIAS (Case 5)

The commonest arrhythmia in old age is atrial fibrillation. In many elderly patients the ventricular response is not fast and the patient does not require treatment. When, however, there is a fast ventricular response digoxin remains useful. But, the window between therapeutic activity and toxicity is small, and even smaller in elderly people with impaired renal function (Case 7). There is also some evidence that the elderly may be more sensitive to the toxic effects of digoxin in terms of malignant arrhythmias. It may be better to use low dose digoxin combined with low dose verapamil to treat fast atrial fibrillation and at the same time avoid adverse drug effects. Fast atrial fibrillation may be due to hyperthyroidism, recurrent pulmonary emboli, rheumatic heart disease, cardiac amyloid, as well as coronary artery disease. These conditions should be sought and treated in their own right. It may also occur as a non-specific entity. Cerebral embolism with resultant cerebral infarction (Chapter 8) and "stroke" are more common in subjects with atrial fibrillation. Anticoagulants are indicated if there is clear evidence of embolism, and should be continued indefinitely.

The elderly heart is subject to numerous brady- and tachy-arrhythmias. The pure tachyarrhythmias may or may not produce symptoms depending on the ventricular rate. Paroxysms of atrial flutter or fibrillation should be treated in the same way as persistent atrial fibrillation. The transient arrhythmias are only diagnosed by 24 hour ambulatory monitoring (Holter) and it has proved difficult to relate the arrhythmias to symptoms. Symptomatic patients with tachyarrhythmias should be treated. The bradyarrhythmias are much more significant in terms of producing symptoms. Persistent bradycardia with rates of less than 50 beats per minute usually present as Stokes–Adams attacks on exercise and a standard 12 lead ECG usually proves the diagnosis. All patients, whatever their age and also probably whatever their condition, with complete or second (Mobitz type II) degree heart block should be treated urgently by pacemaker implantation. This should be carried out at a recognised centre where other electrophysiological investigations may be performed, as appropriate, and the correct type of pacemaker fitted. Patients must be kept under regular review by the pacemaker centre. It is worth emphasising that second degree atrial ventricular block can no longer be considered as a benign arrhythmia.

A particular arrhythmia almost confined to elderly patients is the bradycardia–tachycardia syndrome associated with intrinsic sinus node dysfunction, the "sick sinus syndrome" (Case 5). The patient suffers episodic tachyarrhythmias with multiple extrasystoles. Sustained tachycardia causes symptoms. Unfortunately the tachyarrhythmias are interspersed with occasional brady-arrhythmias. The bradyarrhythmic episodes may not be suspected by the clinician who may use anti-arrhythmics to suppress the tachyarrhythmia and extrasystoles. "Whilst man cannot live by extrasystoles alone they are very helpful when the underlying rhythm may be very slow!" This syndrome should always be treated by pacemaker insertion followed by drug suppression of tachyarrhythmias.

POSTURAL HYPOTENSION

Changing from the lying to the sitting position to standing leads to the pooling of approximately half a litre of blood within the legs. This blood is not available to the systemic circulation and if no compensation is made, leads to a drop in cerebral perfusion. The main compensatory mechanisms are reflex in origin and involve increases in heart rate and peripheral resistance and dilatation of cerebral arterioles. These are mediated by a complex and integrated mechanism involving sensory afferents and autonomic and neuroendocrine efferents. Elderly people are more likely to have deficiencies in this reflex arc because of changes in the autonomic nervous system. Additional causes are usually involved (Table 10.6) and in an individual patient several of these may be present.

The management of postural hypotension involves accurate diagnosis—a drop in systolic blood pressure of 20 mm or more, plus or minus a drop in diastolic blood pressure of 10 mm or more on standing for 2 minutes. Some patients may be symptomatic approximately 1 hour after meals (post-prandial hypotension) if there is a diversion of blood to the gastrointestinal tract during active absorption or during exercise due to diversion of blood to skeletal muscles. Measurement of the blood pressure at appropriate times will confirm the diagnosis. Specific treatment depends on

Table 10.6   Contributing factors associated with postural hypotension and syncope in old age

Environmental	*Cardiovascular*
Immobility/recumbency	Myocardial infarction
Hot weather/bath	Arrhythmias
Exercise	Aortic stenosis
Post-prandial	Mitral valve prolapse
Blood volume	*Metabolic*
Dehydration	Diabetes mellitus
Hyponatraemia	Addison's disease
Varicose veins	Thyrotoxicosis
Hypokalaemia	Hypopituitarism
Haemorrhage	Myxoedema
Anaemia (B_{12})	Porphyria
Physiological	*Drug*
Cough	Antihypertensives
Micturition	Phenothiazines
Defaecation	Tranquillisers
Isometric exercise	Tricyclic antidepressants
Pyrexia	Alcohol
Rectal examination	Levodopa

removal of precipitating or potentiating causes (Table 10.6). To the minority who do not respond to these measures, full waist-length graduated elastic stockings are of benefit, but they can be difficult to put on. Elevation of the head of the bed during the night prevents nocturnal diuresis. Drugs in the main work by producing hypertension or cause fluid and electrolyte retention, so are of little benefit. Practical advice regarding graduated changes in position, particularly on rising first thing in the morning, may prove to be very helpful. Any method by which the patient's general physical fitness can be improved will help the syndrome. Postural hypotension prolongs rehabilitation after bed rest and saps the elderly patient's confidence and morale. Prevention is the key.

HEART VALVES (Case 10)

Aortic Valve

Valves on the left side of the heart (aortic and mitral) are subject to wear and tear over time as well as diseases specific for old age.

Fibrosis and calcification of the aortic valve and its supporting tissue is very common (aortic sclerosis) and gives rise to an aortic systolic murmur. With time, this may progress to aortic stenosis and the development of a significant gradient across the valve. This can be assessed by echocardiography and continuous wave Doppler. Therefore, while the diagnosis of uncomplicated aortic sclerosis does not require treatment, it should not be viewed with complacency. These patients should be monitored at regular intervals and as soon as the gradient becomes significant should be referred for cardiothoracic assessment.

Acute aortic incompetence is due to aortic dissection or bacterial endocarditis. Emergency surgery is the only treatment. Elderly patients do well with aortic valve replacement though the immediate operative mortality is somewhat higher than in younger patients. The main prognostic features relate to left ventricular function and coronary artery disease.

Mitral Valve (Case 10)

Mitral stenosis resulting from early life rheumatic fever rarely presents in old age. Mitral regurgitation (Case 10) may be functional when associated with AV dilatation during severe heart failure. Alternatively it may be related to mitral annular calcification which is revealed by plain radiography. This condition probably affects 1% of elderly people and is a risk factor for subsequent stroke.

Endocarditis

Infective endocarditis in the absence of prosthetic valves is now rarely seen in the developed world in patients under the age of 60 years. The presentation of subacute bacterial endocarditis in elderly patients may be predominately non-cardiac—weight loss, general malaise, anaemia, confusion or the complications of embolisation. A change in heart murmurs may be a clue. Pyrexia may or may not be a feature. Echocardiographic investigation is very helpful and in particular transoesophageal echocardiography may reveal valve vegetations. A high index of suspicion is required for this condition and at least six blood cultures over 48 hours should be carried out. As many patients have been exposed to antibiotics prior to the diagnosis, a precise microbiological assessment is required. Antibiotic prophylaxis should not be forgotten in elderly patients with valve lesions, and the increasing number of dentate subjects must be remembered as a group at particular risk from endocarditis.

BLOOD PRESSURE IN OLD AGE (Cases 2 and 7)

In young and middle-aged adults, increased blood pressure is associated with cardiovascular morbidity and increased mortality and this hazard continues up to the age of 80 years. The higher the blood pressure the greater the risk. Pharmacological lowering of blood pressure in these patients reduces some complications (stroke, cardiac failure, angina) but is much less effective with other complications (myocardial infarct). As a result of atherosclerosis and other factors in Western man, the average blood pressure increases with increasing age. This trend continues up to an age of about 85–90 years of age and then levels off or actually decreases. This latter phenomenon may be due to selective survival. The association, however, between increasing blood pressure and morbidity/mortality becomes less tight and may disappear beyond the age of 80 years. Somewhat paradoxically, the higher the blood pressure beyond this age the better the survival! But there is no doubt that treatment up to this age is effective though evidence of benefit after this age is conflicting.

Who to Treat?

Firstly, the younger old (retirement to 75 years of age) are more likely to benefit from treatment and to suffer less adverse drug effects than the older old (more than 85 years of age). Patients with significant degrees of symptomatic end organ failure (heart failure, angina, renal impairment, cerebral haemorrhage) should be seriously considered for treatment. The obese, smokers, alcohol abusers and the indolent should be given suitable advice and reassessed. If they are unable to comply with lifestyle modification they are unlikely to be good drug compliers and the benefits of treatment will be small compared with the hazard of smoking and obesity. A blood pressure of 160/90 defines hypertension according to the World Health Organisation (WHO). In elderly asymptomatic patients perhaps slightly higher levels would be allowed before commencing treatment. The question sometimes arises "should patients on long-term hypotensives have their drugs withdrawn?" There is no doubt that some previously hypertensive patients remain normotensive on drug withdrawal and some do not. Good studies are not available and at present it is probably best to continue treatment in the absence of significant adverse drug effects. Common sense suggests that if drugs are to be withdrawn they should be tailed off while monitoring blood pressure.

Antihypertensive Agents

It is important to ensure compliance by not giving drugs which render asymptomatic patients symptomatic. A very low dose of a thiazide diuretic (bendrofluazide 2.5 mg daily) would be the first step. This is just as effective an antihypertensive as a larger dose, and is much less likely to give rise to metabolic and other side effects. If a diuretic on its own is not successful in lowering blood pressure to below 160/90, an ACE inhibitor should be introduced, with the usual precautions (initial low dose, check renal function), the dose being titrated against the response in blood pressure. Very rarely is it necessary to add third line antihypertensives such as beta-adrenergic receptor blocking agents, calcium channel antagonists or direct arterial vasodilators. These latter drugs cause significant adverse effects in elderly patients.

PERIPHERAL VASCULAR DISEASE

The generalised atherosclerosis responsible for most cardiovascular disease also affects the aorta and the major peripheral arteries, particularly those supplying the lower limb. In this case the two major risk factors are cigarette smoking and diabetes mellitus. The former affects larger more proximal vessels whilst the latter mainly affects smaller and more distal blood vessels. The management of peripheral vascular disease in diabetics is covered in Chapter 13.

As mentioned earlier in this chapter, unfolding of the aortic arch is often seen on routine chest radiography. While this, in itself, is unimportant, intimal tears with resulting dissecting aneurysms may occur. These are associated with severe pain, and rupture may occur. This is not a uncommon cause of sudden death in the elderly and urgent surgery is needed if the patient is to survive such an episode. It has been suggested that screening older people at the age of 75 years, by abdominal radiography and, if indicated, ultrasonography, may be a cost-effective exercise, in that it is better to electively replace a dilated abdominal aorta than to have to attempt surgery after rupture has occurred.

Large vessel arterial disease of the lower limbs leads to ischaemia on exercise. Classically this presents as intermittent claudication. However, the relationship of symptoms of claudication to degree of occlusion is somewhat loose. Many patients seem to unconsciously limit their exercise to avoid the symptom and do not complain. Treatment after surgical assessment should be offered at an early stage. With suitable patients the results are encouraging. However, it must be recalled that the peripheral vessels reflect the coronary arteries and these patients have considerable macrovascular mortality (myocardial infarctions and strokes). Indeed improving exercise ability by increasing the blood supply to the legs may sometimes result in the onset of angina and the need to improve the myocardial blood supply.

Sudden blockage of a major artery is an emergency and requires urgent surgical referral. If endarterectomy cannot be undertaken or is unsuccessful, amputation usually will be needed. To achieve the best result the patient should be introduced to the rehabilitation team and counselled before his operation, if this is possible. But, surgery should not be delayed for this reason as any delay will increase the toxic complications of early gangrene (acidosis, hyperkalaemia, renal failure). The use of a temporary pylon at a very early stage postoperatively will boost morale and encourage independence. However, in some individuals it becomes obvious that they will not progress with a prosthesis and a relatively early decision to aim for wheelchair independence is best taken. This decision must be taken by the full rehabilitation team which should include the patient and an experienced physiotherapist.

CHAPTER 11   The ageing lung

AGEING AND VENTILATION

In healthy young people the levels of oxygen (O_2) and carbon dioxide (CO_2) in the arterial blood are kept within narrow limits. Any fall in O_2 or rise in CO_2 results in a rapid increase in the depth and rate of respiration. With ageing there is a gradual deterioration in the efficiency of this mechanism. Degenerative changes occur in the cells of the ventilatory centres in the brain stem, and the O_2 receptors in the carotid and aortic bodies, so that there is a diminished response to changes in these gases.

The thoracic cage becomes more rigid, as we age, due to calcification of costal cartilage and degeneration of the joints articulating ribs with dorsal vertebrae together with wasting of the intercostal muscles and the diaphragm. Compounding these changes, the structure of the connective tissue within the lung is modified so that collagen stiffens and lung elasticity falls. The airways become "floppy" and tend to collapse on expiration.

The physiological consequences of these changes are that when old people breathe out the elastic recoil pressure is lower so airflow is also lower. Air "trapped" in the lung is increased. Inspiration is not affected (Table 11.1 and Figure 11.1).

PRACTICAL CONSEQUENCES

The increased rigidity of the thoracic cage together with the loss of elasticity of lung tissue means that old people are more likely to become breathless with less exertion than the young, though this, in the absence of pathology, should not limit appropriate exercise. Because respiratory excursion and force is diminished the breath sounds, on auscultation, are softer and abnormal sounds are more difficult to detect when lung disease exists. Coughing is less effective so that bronchial secretions tend to accumulate, particu-

Table 11.1   Age changes in lung function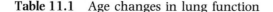

Static volumes	Total lung capacity (TLC)	Unchanged
	Vital capacity	Decreased
	Closing volume	Increased
	Functional residual capacity	Increased
	Residual volume	Increased
Dynamic volumes	Forced expiratory volume (FEV$_1$)	Decreased
	Maximum breathing capacity (MBC)	Decreased
	Peak expiratory flow rate (PEFR)	Decreased

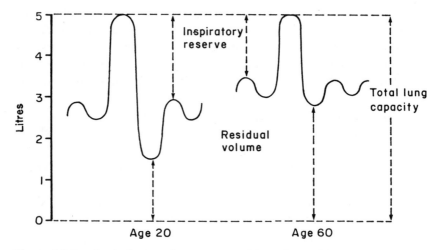

Figure 11.1   Static lung volume at age 20 and age 60

larly when the individual is recumbent. The presence of basal crepitations is therefore of less value as a physical sign than it is in the younger patient and should be ignored unless there is other evidence of a pathological cause (Chapter 10). Lung function tests may be difficult to interpret for their pattern in the elderly is similar to that found in the younger patient with obstructed airways. Interpretation requires that the age of the patient be taken into account. Finally a reduced response to anoxia or hypercapnia (high CO_2 level) means that under conditions of stress, such as a chest infection, old people are more likely to develop a blood gas imbalance leading to drowsiness, confusion and increased mortality.

OBSTRUCTIVE SYNDROMES (Cases 7 and 9)

The three major obstructive syndromes are chronic bronchitis, emphysema and asthma. An attempt to differentiate between these three conditions often is not made, and the three are lumped together under the heading of chronic obstructive airways disease (COAD).

Simple chronic bronchitis is defined by the British Medical Research Council as an increase in the volume of sputum sufficent to cause expectoration on most days during three successive months for more than two successive years, with the exclusion of focal causes such as bronchiectasis. *Complicated chronic bronchitis* refers to the development of infective exacerbations or of airways obstruction giving rise to shortness of breath. The prevalence of chronic bronchitis, as defined, in a recent survey in the New Forest area of Hampshire was 16.4%; it did not increase with increasing age and was commoner amongst smokers. As in all other age groups, women are less affected than men, a fact probably related to their smoking habits; this may change in the future.

The World Health Organisation (WHO) defines *emphysema* as a condition of the lungs characterised by an increase beyond the normal size of the air space distal to the terminal bronchioles brought about by destruction of their walls. The patient with primary emphysema tends to be younger than the one with more classical chronic bronchitis. Diagnosis of the condition is difficult, since damage to this part of the air space may be the result of other respiratory disease, particularly infections. Emphysema is, therefore, a common complication of other lung diseases. Characteristically, the emphysematous patient complains of breathlessness, often at rest, in the absence of significant bronchial secretion. Most cases occur in very heavy cigarette smokers. Cigarette smoke promotes neutrophil and macrophage elastase and the protective effects of antitrypsin may be negated or antitrypsin itself destroyed. The distinction between chronic bronchitis and emphysema is artificial in that most patients, to a greater or lesser extent, exhibit features of both disorders.

Asthma is a disease characterised by a variable resistance in the airways which may disappear either spontaneously or as a result of treatment. It used to be thought that asthma was a disease primarily affecting young people, but, during the last 20 years, its high prevalence in the elderly as a discrete entity has been recognised and, indeed, it may arise for the first time in the very old.

Unfortunately, it seems that the elderly are more likely to develop infective complications with asthma, which makes it difficult to distinguish from chronic bronchitis with airways obstruction. Failure to diagnose the condition has serious consequences in that a patient is denied the intensive therapy which often is effective in controlling symptoms. Characteristic features include a family history of asthma or a previous history of asthma as a child. Symptoms may be provoked by exercise. Wheezing may be noticed by the spouse in the early hours of the morning, or the patient wake with cough. The latter symptoms are associated with early morning depression of respiratory function ("early morning dips").

MANAGEMENT OF CHRONIC OBSTRUCTIVE SYNDROMES

Every effort should be made to stop patients with chronic bronchitis from smoking. This will not influence the progressive downhill nature of the disease, but will reduce the liability to recurrent infections, which, when they occur, should be treated with a broad spectrum antibiotic. Trimethoprim and co-amoxiclav are drugs of first choice for elderly patients with community acquired infections.

BRONCHODILATORS

Inhaled beta-adrenoceptor agonists such as salbutamol or terbutaline are of obvious benefit where there is bronchospasm. They are safe and effective and may be given as nebulised inhalations, or administered by "spacers" or other volume devices. Some elderly find inhalers difficult to use and instruction in their use is mandatory. One approach is to demonstrate the mode of use and then get patients to practise, under supervision, using a "dummy" inhaler containing an inert substance until they have become proficient.

Non-selective adrenoceptor stimulants such as ephedrine are no longer used. Theophylline, in sustained release form, is a useful addition to beta-adrenoceptor agonists. Corticosteroids may sometimes need to be used to help control asthma. They are best given in an inhaled form since this reduces the risk of systemic effects. Aerosol forms used in conjunction with a beta-adrenoceptor agonist represent a real advance in the management of asthma in some older people. Their addition to the inhaler regime may improve exercise tolerance markedly, enabling an individual, for instance, to play golf without resorting to the use of an inhaler. Thrush (oropharyngeal candidiasis) occurs in some patients but responds to treatment with antifungal agents and its incidence can be controlled by using a spacer device or reducing the dose or frequency of dosage of the corticosteroid.

Antihistamines may be used occasionally if hay fever or vasomotor rhinitis is troublesome. The newer antihistamines, such as astemizole, are particularly useful as they hardly penetrate the blood–brain barrier, cause fewer adverse reactions and have a once daily dosage.

Long-term oxygen therapy, up to 18 hours a day, is useful in anoxic COAD patients of any age. Oxygen concentrators are economical, easily used and safer alternatives to cylinders.

RESTRICTIVE SYNDROMES

The term covers a number of syndromes with a characteristic ventilatory function pattern (Table 11.2). The vital capacity is markedly reduced, but measures of airways obstruction are relatively normal. The patient usually complains of breathlessness on exertion rather than at rest, and although extremely dyspnoeic is quite pink in colour. The production of sputum in these syndromes is unusual. A great number of diseases are known to produce restrictive syndromes, but in the elderly, left ventricular failure in both sexes and rheumatoid arthritis in females account for the majority. Patients with restrictive syndromes do not usually retain CO_2 to any great extent except terminally, so domiciliary oxygen given intermittently is safe and may give considerable symptomatic relief. Bronchodilators are usually inappropriate though steroids may be worth a trial.

PNEUMONIA (Cases 2 and 7)

Pneumonia is classically known as "the old man's friend", since it is a common and often terminal event in old people. Reasons for this include an impaired cough mechanism, impaired local immunological defences, and the frequent association of diseases predisposing to respiratory infection such as cardiac and renal failure. This, however, does not mean that pneumonia should not

Table 11.2 Conditions associated with restrictive syndromes

Left ventricular failure	Idiopathic fibrosis
Fibrosing alveolitis	Systemic lupus erythematosus
Rheumatoid lung	Drugs
Sarcoidosis	Ankylosing spondylitis
Severe kyphoscoliosis	

be treated, but that careful assessment of the patient should be undertaken before treatment is begun. Ethical factors need to be weighed against the patient's known quality of life; his wishes, if he is able to express these clearly (testamentary capacity); the opinion of his general practitioner, and perhaps his spouse or caring relative. Diagnosis, moreover, may be difficult for the usual signs such as cough, sputum, fever and chest pain may be absent. Non-specific features such as falls, heart failure, confusion or reduced mobility are common. A raised respiratory rate above 28/min may be the most useful indication preceding other physical signs or radiological change by as much as 48 hours. Some elderly patients suffer from recurrent bouts of pneumonia (bronchopneumonia). Table 11.3 lists some of the common causes.

Although some cases of pneumonia in the elderly are treated adequately and successfully at home, many patients will undoubtedly benefit from skilled nursing which can be constantly available within the hospital. A suitable broad spectrum bactericidal antibiotic should be chosen. Unfortunately, it is not usually expedient to await the results of sputum and/or blood cultures, although it is wise to obtain specimens prior to antibiotic therapy so that this can be changed later in the light of bacterial sensitivity. Persistent

Table 11.3 Causes of recurrent pneumonia

Obstruction
  carcinoma
  foreign body
Bronchiectasis
Pulmonary abscess
Tuberculosis
Repeated aspiration
  debility
  dysphagia
  post-anaesthesia
  gastro-oesophageal reflux

or recurrent pneumonia or an infection acquired in hospital (nosocomial) always requires bacteriological investigation and the patient treated with a cephalosporin until the results of this are available. Antibiotics should be continued until symptoms and signs have regressed. They may need to be continued for longer than in the younger patient since recovery is slower in old age. Monitoring of the respiratory rate may be helpful and should be continued after antibiotics have been stopped. An increase in rate may then indicate recurrence. Anoxia can be treated with oxygen therapy; if there is any evidence of pre-existing long-standing lung disease this should be in a low concentration, i.e. 28%. Dehydration, preferably, should be prevented, but this is often difficult as these ill patients are reluctant to drink and dehydration is present on admission. If necessary, intravenous fluids should be administered, but great care must be taken to ensure that congestive cardiac failure is not precipitated.

Similarly, consideration should be given to the nutritional requirements of the patient, since the illness is likely to cause severe under-nutrition and steps must be taken to counteract this. The dietitian has an important part to play in this and enteral feeding may need to be considered in the very ill. This aspect of the management of serious illness in the elderly is frequently neglected.

TUBERCULOSIS

While modern antituberculous drugs have reduced the incidence of tuberculosis in the population at large, the condition remains relatively common in the elderly population. The reasons for this are that patients may have contracted the disease in their youth, and that diminished immunological defences accompanying ageing and ill health may allow a quiescent lung lesion to become reactivated and break down—post primary tuberculosis.

Tuberculosis may present classically with night sweats, weight loss, cough and haemoptysis. More often, in old age, the patient complains of tiredness, loss of appetite and general vague malaise which may well be attributed to "getting old" or depression by the primary care team.

The diagnosis of pulmonary tuberculosis can be made by identifying the characteristic changes on the chest X-ray. Doubt often exists as to whether the changes are due to quiescent or active disease. Microscopy of a sputum specimen may identify acid fast bacilli, and a sample should be sent for culture. If a sputum specimen cannot be obtained, a laryngeal swab will provide suitable material for microscopy and culture. A further approach is to perform a Mantoux test. Unfortunately, immunological changes often mean that even with active tuberculosis a skin test using 5 units of tuberculin PPD may be negative. Where this happens repeating the test with 250 units will usually produce a skin response. If despite this the reaction is negative, a tuberculous infection is most unlikely. A positive reaction means that the patient either has active tuberculosis or has had it in the past. Serial chest X-rays taken at intervals of 2 months will enable the condition to be monitored, and changes in the lesion(s) will confirm activity.

Initial treatment of post-primary tuberculosis in elderly patients should be ethambutol, pyrazinamide, rifampacin and isoniazid for 2 months, or longer (until the result of drug sensitivity testing is known), reducing this to isoniazid with rifampacin for a further 4 months.

One of the problems in the management of tuberculosis in old age is that it may persist unrecognised for years. This means that other members of the household (particularly children) are at risk of infection while the disease itself may have reached a very advanced stage before it is detected in the patient. A chest X-ray is mandatory, therefore, if there is the slightest possibility of there being tuberculosis. This is particularly important if the patient is going into an old people's home or a hospital. There may also be problems of drug compliance. Inadequate medication results not only in the progession of the disease, but also in the development of resistant organisms. The doctor, health visitor or district nurse should keep a close watch on drug intake if this is to be avoided.

MALIGNANT DISEASE (Case 9)

Lung cancer has a peak incidence in the over-70s with a male preponderance. Unfortunately because of changes in smoking habits some 40–50 years ago, women are rapidly catching up. The prevalence of different tumour types is given in Table 11.4.

Symptoms may be due to the tumour itself (cough, haemoptysis, pain), local (pleural effusion, superior vena caval obstruction) or distant metastases (bone pain, cerebral space occupying lesion, hepatic infiltration). Occasionally the patient is asymptomatic and the tumour is seen on a routine chest X-ray.

Table 11.4   Tumour types

Squamous	35%
Small cell	20%
Adenocarcinoma	25%
Others/mixed/large cell	20%

Investigation

The objective here is to establish a diagnosis, including cell type, and whether the disease is extensive or limited. Sputum cytology is unreliable (and unhelpful) in the elderly because many atypical cells are found which do not necessarily represent malignant change. Radiography (including CT) of chest, bones and brain easily establishes the extent of the disease. Bronchoscopy is not only useful for diagnosis and cell typing but also helpful in assessing the suitability of various treatment options, including surgery.

Management

If surgery is contemplated, and too often it is not in elderly patients, histology must confirm that it is not a small cell type. Obviously the patient must have sufficient cardiac and respiratory reserve to cope with a possible pneumonectomy. In appropriate cases, surgery can be extremely effective achieving up to a 40% five year survival. Direct surgery is not an option in the presence of metastatic disease either local or distant.

Radiotherapy may be curative in some patients who are unfit for surgery, but it is also valuable as a palliative treatment for superior vena caval obstruction, local or distant bone pain, and troublesome haemoptysis. Laser therapy is an alternative treatment for haemoptysis and for local bronchial obstruction. An alternative procedure for the latter condition might be bronchoscopic stenting under a local anaesthetic.

Small cell tumours of the bronchus if localised at diagnosis may have a long disease free interval following intravenous chemotherapy. Extensive disease may be palliated with oral drugs such as etoposide. This chemotherapeutic agent is well tolerated with minimal side effects. The role of chemotherapy for squamous carcinoma and adenocarcinoma is still in doubt. Such patients should be referred to local centres performing Phase II drug studies. Too often the elderly are excluded from such assessments.

THROMBOEMBOLIC DISEASE

Pulmonary embolism is a common occurrence in the hospitalised elderly; it is a cause of death in about 12%. Diagnosis may be difficult and is often made at autopsy as an incidental finding. The classical triad of pleuritic chest pain, haemoptysis and dyspnoea is often absent. The presentation is less dramatic though there are usually signs and symptoms indicative of a cardiorespiratory problem. These include breathlessness, cough with sputum production, and often some chest pain or discomfort. On examination there is tachypnoea and moist sounds are heard on auscultation. A diagnosis of congestive cardiac failure is often erroneously made. Alternatively the patient may become confused (Chapter 9) or his general condition deteriorate for no obvious reason. Examination of the chest may reveal diminished breath sounds and coarse crepitations over a lung segment, a pleural friction rub or signs of a pleural effusion; a chest X-ray may show an area of lung collapse or obliteration of a costophrenic angle, suggesting a small pleural effusion. However, none of these signs may be present and a search must be made for evidence of venous thrombosis as a probable source of the embolus. Possible predisposing factors for peripheral vein thrombosis (Table 11.5) are present in three-quarters of patients confirmed as having pulmonary embolism and the finding of any of these should arouse suspicion of the diagnosis. Commonly thrombosis develops in the deep leg veins (Case 4), and local tenderness and lower limb oedema may be present. The clinical signs, though, are often minimal and may be easily missed. The differential diagnosis of pulmonary embolism is one that should always be kept in mind when the condition of an elderly patient in hospital deteriorates. A definitive diagnosis may be made by performing a ventilation–perfusion lung scan. This is well tolerated by elderly patients and has a high degree of sensitivity though the specificity is variable.

Medical and nursing staff should aim at preventing deep vein thrombosis. Old people are at increased risk of this if they are bedfast, or kept sitting in a chair all day. They should be encouraged to walk, even if this requires help from a member of staff. Venous stasis should be kept to a minimum using graded pressure stockings

Table 11.5 Risk factors for venous thrombosis (in addition to immobility)

Moderate risk	Extreme old age
	Gross obesity
	Post-general surgery
	Cardiac/respiratory failure
	Malignancy
	Major trauma/burns
High risk	Lower limb fracture
	Abdominal surgery
	Hemiplegia (rule out haemorrhage)
	Lower limb amputation

(Chapter 10). All elderly patients admitted to hospital should be assessed for risk factors (Table 11.5). Low risk patients only require rapid mobilisation. Most patients with moderate and all those at high risk require additional prophylaxis with low dose subcutaneous heparin which should be maintained until the patient is fully mobile or discharged. Once thrombosis and/or pulmonary embolism has occurred anticoagulants should be given and patients kept on a maintenance dose for a period of 3 to 6 months after their discharge. Other supportive measures include relief of pain, administration of oxygen and treatment of concomitant complications such as infection, faecal impaction (Chapter 14), heart failure and malignant disease.

FURTHER READING

Seaton, A., Seaton, D. and Leitch, A.G. (ed) (1989). *Crofton and Douglas's Respiratory Diseases*. London: Blackwell Scientific Publications.

Thromboembolic Risk Factors (THRIFT) Consensus Group (1992). *Risk of and prophylaxis in hospital patients*. British Medical Journal **305**: 567–573.

CHAPTER 12   The gastrointestinal tract and anaemia

ALIMENTARY DISEASE

Mouth and Teeth

Some of the problems relating to nutrition have already been mentioned in Chapter 6 but the state of the mouth and teeth may also have an important influence in this area. On average denture wearers chew only one-sixth as well as young dentate adults, but take twice as long. Good dental care of the elderly, therefore, is important but is often neglected. Carious and broken teeth or ill-fitting dentures are uncomfortable and may give rise to oral ulceration as well as inefficient mastication. As the majority of the elderly are edentulous, most of the treatment relates to the stomatognathic changes which occur; consequently, denture cleaning, relining, rebasing, easing and repairing should be considered in all those who wear false teeth. It should be remembered that some elderly people are sensitive to modern plastics used in the manufacture of false teeth, so that repairing and refitting old dentures may be better than making new sets.

It is likely in the future that many more old people will have at least some of their own teeth. This is due to the reduction in the prevalence of dental caries which has occurred as a result of the wider use of fluorine. It is now estimated that over one-third of the over-75s and two-thirds of the over-65s will be dentate in the year 1998. Continuing dental care will therefore be necessary for a larger proportion of the population. This may pose problems to those who are housebound and the amount of domiciliary dentistry needed is likely to increase. Dental surgeries will need to be accessible to the frailer and disabled patient, while dentists will need to have a greater knowledge of the pathology of ageing.

Many old people complain of a sore tongue or mouth ulcers. While these may be related to dental trauma (see above), other causes such as vitamin deficiency (Chapter 6), anaemia (this chapter) and other blood diseases, as well as aphthous ulceration and infection may occur. Treatment should be directed to the cause.

Aphthous ulceration is painful and causes considerable discomfort. While the ulcers usually heal spontaneously they may be slow to do so, interfering with denture wearing and reducing food intake. Treatment with low dose hydrocortisone pellets (Corlan) or local insufflation of sodium cromoglycate will aid healing and relieve symptoms.

A sore tongue may be associated with drug therapy, neurosis, depressive illness or infection. Perhaps the commonest infection is the fungus, monilia (*Candida albicans*), commonly known as thrush. It should always be suspected if white patches are seen on the tongue, throat or buccal mucosa. Diagnosis is confirmed by identification of characteristic hyphae on microscopy, or by culture of the lesion and the rapid response to local applications of nystatin given in the form of drops or lozenges. The condition is common in those with severe debility, diabetes mellitus or in infections that have been treated with broad spectrum antibiotics, and in patients using corticosteroid inhalers (Chapter 11). The condition must be differentiated from leukoplakia, a condition which is potentially neoplastic, particularly if it affects the tongue. A fungal infection may be apparently resistant to treatment in some patients and progress to chronic hyperplastic candidiasis. This is more likely in permanent denture wearers, particularly if they smoke or are diabetic. Cleaning dentures or teeth twice daily may help to cure the condition and prevent its recurrence. Treatment with nystatin should continue until the symptoms and signs of the disease have disappeared.

Dysphagia (Cases 3 and 10)

Difficulty in swallowing usually is associated with lesions of the oesophagus. However, a careful history is helpful in elucidating the problem and defining what it is meant by the complaint. Ill-fitting dentures give rise to inefficient mastication and difficulty in swallowing the resultant bolus; salivary flow is reduced with ageing, as well as in some diseases, with dehydration and with many drugs, so that the resultant dry mouth is a problem; pharyngeal lesions such as pouches and postcricoid webs also may occur. Whether there is a difference between swallowing solids and liquids or both, and the level at which the difficulty occurs helps define the diagnosis. Neurological lesions (Chapter 8), particularly "strokes" with or without pseudobulbar palsy, cause dysphagia due to the effect they have on the innervation and coordination of the muscles of the oropharynx (Case 3). In these circumstances a speech therapist may be able to help with breathing and feeding advice.

Damage to the wall of the oesophagus by acid reflux may cause narrowing (benign stricture) with resultant dysphagia, the patient usually being able to indicate the level at which food "sticks". It can be treated by mechanical dilatation, but with repeated dilatation the risk of rupture increases. Cancer of the oesophagus (Case 10) causing a malignant stricture, pressure from enlarged mediastinal glands or tumours of the lung also cause dysphagia with a pattern similar to that resulting from a benign stricture. The prospect of slow death by starvation, in these latter conditions is so appalling that the advice of a surgeon should be sought, no matter how old or frail the patient. Palliative measures may secure a less unpleasant death.

External pressure also may be caused by an enlarged left atrium or dilated arteriosclerotic blood vessel such as the aorta or innominate artery. When this happens no treatment apart from reassurance is necessary.

Dysphagia should be investigated by barium swallow and endoscopy. The former, in some old patients, may show abnormal oesophageal contractions. The appearance has been called "corkscrew oesophagus" and has been attributed to ageing (presbyoesophagus). In this condition, the lower oesophageal sphincter does not relax in coordination with the peristaltic wave, which itself may be weak, infrequent and unrelated to swallowing. Nonperistaltic contractions (tertiary contractions) occur and delayed emptying may result in dilatation of the oesophagus. The clinical significance of this is doubtful. However, disorders of oesophageal motility may be intermittent and barium swallow and endoscopy may be normal. In these cases 24 hour oesophageal motility studies, using manometry, should be undertaken. This may show diffuse oesophageal spasm with high amplitude, aperistaltic, prolonged contractions associated with normal lower oesophageal sphincter relaxation. These may cause not only dysphagia but also non-cardiac chest pain. The condition responds to treatment with nifedipine, the effect of which is dose dependent.

Gastro-oesophageal Reflux Disease (GORD)

Well over half of all elderly people have reflux oesophagitis and/or hiatus hernia though not all have symptoms. The symptoms are associated with regurgitation of stomach contents or acid and tend to occur when lying down or bending over. They include dysphagia, dyspepsia, vomiting, heartburn, and chest pain, which may be difficult to differentiate from angina due to myocardial ischaemia occurring at rest. Respiratory symptoms (cough, hoarseness, wheezing) are common, and are due to recurrent episodes of aspiration. Anaemia may result from persistent occult blood loss, though hiatus hernia is so common in old people that other causes of anaemia should be sought before concluding that this is responsible. Oesophageal reflux is usually due to dysfunction of the lower oesophageal sphincter, most episodes occurring when the sphincter relaxes. The prevalence of hiatus hernia rises with age and leads to reflux, probably because the sphincter is lifted out of the abdominal cavity, thereby making it incompetent. Smoking, alcohol and obesity all reduce sphincter pressure and increase reflux.

Diagnosis of reflux oesophagitis is confirmed by endoscopy, while a hiatus hernia can be demonstrated by a barium swallow. Treatment is aimed at reducing reflux and neutralising the effects of acid either by lining the lower oesophageal mucosa with an antacid or De-Nol and, if necessary, combining this with an H_2 receptor blocker. Measures to reduce reflux include raising the head of the bed (propping the patient up with pillows increases abdominal pressure and thereby reflux); weight reduction; eating small meals to reduce gastric distension; stopping smoking; and restricting alcohol intake. Motility modifying drugs (dopamine agonists) may also help by increasing lower oesophageal sphincter tone and peristalsis. If medical measures fail or the symptoms relapse, surgery may be necessary. The results of this are good and the decision to operate should be based upon the severity of the symptoms, and the general medical condition of the patient rather than his age.

Peptic Ulcer (Case 1)

Duodenal and gastric ulcers reach a peak incidence in middle age but remain sufficiently common in old age to cause a lot of trouble (about 20% peptic ulcers occur in the elderly). They may present in a variety of ways, particularly with general malaise, anorexia, dyspepsia, vomiting, epigastric pain and haemorrhage.

Pain

This symptom is often absent because the elderly may have an increased threshold to painful stimuli and a reduced inflammatory response to tissue injury. Peptic ulceration may thus remain an unsuspected cause of weight loss, anaemia, or even confusion in many old people.

Haemorrhage

This is the most serious complication of peptic ulceration in old age, and, when acute, is associated with high mortality. This is probably the result of the high prevalence of coexistent disease rather than ageing itself. The only way to minimise the risk is to control the haemorrhage as quickly as possible. Bleeding may respond to high dose H_2 antagonists but failure or a second bleed makes operation imperative. In recent years, gastroenterologists have reduced the risk from surgery by cauterising the bleeding vessels during endoscopy. If this is unsuccessful, it should be followed immediately by laparotomy. In situations where local treatment or surgery is deemed inappropriate, there rarely is ethical justification for massive and prolonged blood transfusion as this will only prolong dying rather than save life.

Chronic haemorrhage giving rise to iron deficiency anaemia is also common (see below: hypochromic anaemia), and may sometimes be associated with a giant gastric ulcer; this can only be differentiated from gastric cancer by a biopsy.

Investigation and treatment

Diagnosis, particularly in the case of a giant gastric ulcer, can only be made with certainty by endoscopy (Chapter 3). If adequately premedicated with a benzodiazepine, many old people sleep through the procedure and remember nothing afterwards apart from the unpleasantness of the local anaesthetic throat spray. Chronic gastritis is usually associated with *Helicobacter pylori* (previously *Campylobacter pylori*) infection. Whether *Helicobacter pylori* infection is a cause of peptic ulcer is uncertain, but some evidence suggests that the association is stronger with duodenal than gastric ulcers. Chronic low-grade gastritis and slow bleeding often is due to taking non-steroidal anti-inflammatory drugs (NSAIDs).

Antacids reduce gastric acidity, particularly if they are taken 1 and 3 hours after meals, and still have a part to play in the symptomatic treatment of peptic ulcer. A nocturnal H_2 antagonist is the treatment of choice. They should be continued for 6 weeks and healing confirmed by endoscopy. In the rare case of failure, the proton pump inhibitor, omeprazole, should be given. Cimetidine may cause confusion and interact with other drugs, and ranitidine is to be preferred for elderly patients. *Helicobacter pylori*, if found by accident at biopsy, should be treated with a combination of ampicillin and metronidazole for 2 weeks. Infection should also be sought and treated, if found, in patients with recurrent duodenal ulceration. Sucralfate, the aluminium salt of sulphated sucrose, may help healing and prevent recurrence. It is safe to use, as it is not absorbed, can be given twice daily, and may reduce faecal blood loss associated with NSAIDs. Surgery is only indicated when acute haemorrhage, pyloric stenosis or perforation occur.

Gastric Cancer

The symptoms of this condition also are often vague and ill-defined, varying from a "failure to thrive" to frank depression or even an acute confusional state. The standard explanation is that these symptoms are produced by toxins released by the tumour cells.

Surgery has little effect on the life expectancy of patients with gastric carcinoma, unless the diagnosis is made early, and this is often fortuitous. Symptoms of the tumour itself, such as pain, dysphagia and bleeding, are usually late and too late for more than palliative surgical intervention.

Previous gastric surgery

Any list of elderly patients "at risk" from poor nutrition in the community should include people who have had surgery for peptic ulceration. Alteration of the anatomy or function of the upper alimentary tract can cause malabsorption of a wide range of nutrients, which in the elderly can produce severe weight loss, severe anaemia, and loss of bone mass with an increased risk of fractures. Less specifically, the already decreased resistance to infection is accentuated so that reactivation of a long quiescent focus of pulmonary tuberculosis may occur (Chapter 11).

Complications often develop 20 or 30 years after an operation when the episode has been forgotten by doctor and the patient alike. Failure to identify the problem condemns the patient to chronic ill health and may result in permanent disability.

Malabsorption

Malabsorption may occur in old people, as in any other age group. Causes of this include gluten sensitive enteropathy, diverticula of the duodenum and jejunum, previous gastric surgery and bacterial overgrowth of the duodenum and jejunum. Complex investigation may be necessary to elucidate the problem. The condition is frequently missed, associated weight loss being attributed to a poor diet, but as a dietary deficiency is rare in active old people, any weight loss should be viewed seriously and a cause sought. Treatment should then be directed at the cause. Bacterial overgrowth of the small bowel is a relatively common finding in old age. It may not be associated, always, with diverticula or "blind loops", and does occur in fit active elderly. However, when it leads to malabsorption, it may be reversed by giving long-term treatment with an appropriate antibiotic.

Gallbladder Disease

This occurs in 25% of people over the age of 70 years. It is often asymptomatic, being found at autopsy, having required no treatment, and only causing the occasional episode of flatulence after a heavy meal. When the condition does flare up as bile duct obstruction and inflammation (cholecystitis) it can be very unpleasant, giving rise to severe abdominal pain. It may also present atypically as an acute illness often with confusion and few abdominal symptoms. Mortality bears a direct relationship to the age and disability of the patient.

Recent advances have meant that the need for major abdominal surgery has almost disappeared. Patients with ductal stones and functioning gallbladders can be treated by endoscopic retrograde cholangiopancreatography (ERCP) examination associated with endoscopic papillotomy and removal of obstructing calculi, using lithotripsy or irrigation if necessary. This technique means that the frail and very old can be treated with lower risk and avoids the need for cholecystectomy. Patients with a diseased gallbladder may be treated by one of the newer minimal access surgical procedures—percutaneous stone extraction with gallstone lithotripsy using ultrasonic fragmentation; percutaneous cholecystotomy; or laparoscopic cholecystectomy, which is becoming the treatment of choice. In the best hands the operation takes about 1 hour, and if home care is good, may even be done as day surgery. In over 12 000 cases reviewed from seven European centres there were no deaths, morbidity was very low and the median hospital stay was 3 days.

Bile acids have been used to dissolve stones, but are effective only against cholesterol stones, take many months to work, do not treat the underlying disease and, consequently have a very limited practical application.

Jaundice

Table 12.1 lists the relative percentage frequencies for the major causes of jaundice in elderly hospital patients; the particular importance of drugs as a cause of jaundice should be noted. Many potentially hepatotoxic drugs are in wide general use in geriatric practice. They include the anticonvulsant phenytoin, the tranquillisers such as phenothiazines and the anabolic derivatives of testosterone. A careful drug history must therefore be elicited in all cases of jaundice. This can usefully be supplemented by a careful search around the house, for old people are notorious hoarders and may be taking tablets prescribed many years previously for themselves or for some long dead relative (Chapter 5).

Pancreatic Disease

Chronic pancreatitis is rare in old age but carcinoma of the pancreas seems to be commoner, particularly in men over 75 years, and is increasing in frequency, possibly because of environmental factors, such as smoking, alcohol and coffee intake. Obstructive jaundice, malaise, abdominal pain and depression are common symptoms. Biliary obstruction can be relieved by insertion of a stent at ERCP or by open surgery. The prognosis is extremely poor.

Appendicitis

As with other causes of abdominal pain, the symptoms of appendicitis in the elderly are often mild and poorly localised (Chapter 2). A vague abdominal ache may be attributed to constipation and either ignored or treated with laxatives. Poor tissue resistance results in a rapid evolution from local sepsis to generalised peritonitis so that by the time a doctor is consulted the patient may be moribund. While appendicitis is uncommon in the elderly, diagnosis before peritonitis ensues is essential if a high mortality is to be avoided.

Peritonitis

The classical signs of abdominal pain, tenderness, rigidity, distension and diminished or absent bowel sounds are often missing in elderly patients. In a recent series of older patients the commonest single cause was mesenteric infarction, though perforation of the bowel associated with peptic ulcer, diverticulitis, or intestinal

Table 12.1   Causes of jaundice in the elderly

Condition	Percentage
Cancer of the biliary tract	22
Drugs	21
Calculi in biliary tract	16
Hepatitis	15
Hepatic secondaries	12
Cirrhosis	10
Haemolysis	4

obstruction accounted for more than a third of the cases. The diagnostic accuracy was less than 50%. Tenderness or distension was present in about three-quarters, diminished or absent bowel sounds in half and rigidity in only a third. Abdominal pain was present in less than half but when associated with fever, tachycardia and nausea or vomiting increased the level of diagnositic accuracy. Mortality was 96%.

Diverticular Disease (Case 4)

Almost half the population over 70 years of age have diverticular disease of the colon. The symptoms are usually minimal but complications such as massive haemorrhage, or abscess formation are fairly common. The disease is probably the consequence of the highly refined low-roughage diets taken in Western society. Muscle contraction in the colonic wall is normally used to push faeces along the lumen. When faeces are low in bulk, muscle contraction merely increases the intraluminal pressure which, ultimately, results in the herniation of gut mucosa through areas of weakness in the muscle coat with diverticulum formation.

The condition can be prevented or minimised by increasing the amount of roughage in the diet. Bran is a useful source of roughage; tastes vary, but most patients prefer to take it mixed with ordinary meals, and a dose of one tablespoon up to three times daily is usual.

Cancer of Colon and Rectum

Cancer of the lower alimentary tract sometimes presents dramatically as an acute obstruction or perforation; more often, it results in a gradual deterioration in health associated with a change in bowel habit. A sudden change in bowel function may be due to faecal impaction (Chapter 14), but the possibility of cancer should always be considered and, if necessary, excluded by endoscopic or radiological examination.

Ulcerative Colitis, Crohn's Disease, Ischaemic Colitis

Each of these conditions may occur in old age and ischaemic colitis is particularly associated with the ageing process. In the first two conditions the radiological appearance of the barium enema show-ing a loss of the colon's haustral pattern. In ischaemic colitis a "thumb-print" type of indentation is seen in the barium pattern. Confirmation of the diagnosis of Crohn's disease is by biopsy.

Rectal Prolapse

This is a common and very uncomfortable and distressing con-dition. It is frequently found in women and may relate to damage to the anal sphincter which can occur in childbearing; it results in faecal incontinence or soiling. Treatment is aimed   at either restoring anal sphincter tone or reducing the size of the anus by inserting a silver wire. Thereafter, stools must be kept soft and constipation avoided (Chapter 14).

ANAEMIA (Cases 4 and 10)

The prevalence of anaemia depends on the population sample stud-ied, as well as on the haemoglobin level below which anaemia is said to occur. In old age the lower levels of normal for haemoglobin are 13 g/dl for men and 12 g/dl for women. Community surveys show a prevalence of between 5 and 15%, while the prevalence in elderly subjects admitted to hospital is as high as 40%.

Investigation

Investigation should start with a detailed history. Particular points requiring consideration include alimentary symptoms, dietary habits, previous gastrointestinal surgery, and analgesic or steroid intake. A detailed physical examination, including rectal examin-ation, is essential, and where necessary this should be followed by laboratory investigations (Chapter 3). Figure 12.1 details a rational approach to this problem. Investigation also should be governed by whether action will be taken if a test is positive; a surgeon is unlikely to resect a carcinoma in a confused, bedfast and doubly incontinent 95-year-old man, though treatment of his anaemia may improve his confusion and make him more comfortable.

Hypochromic (Microcytic) Anaemia (Case 4)

Iron deficiency anaemia is by far the commonest cause of anaemia in old age; it is occasionally due to dietary deficiency but is much

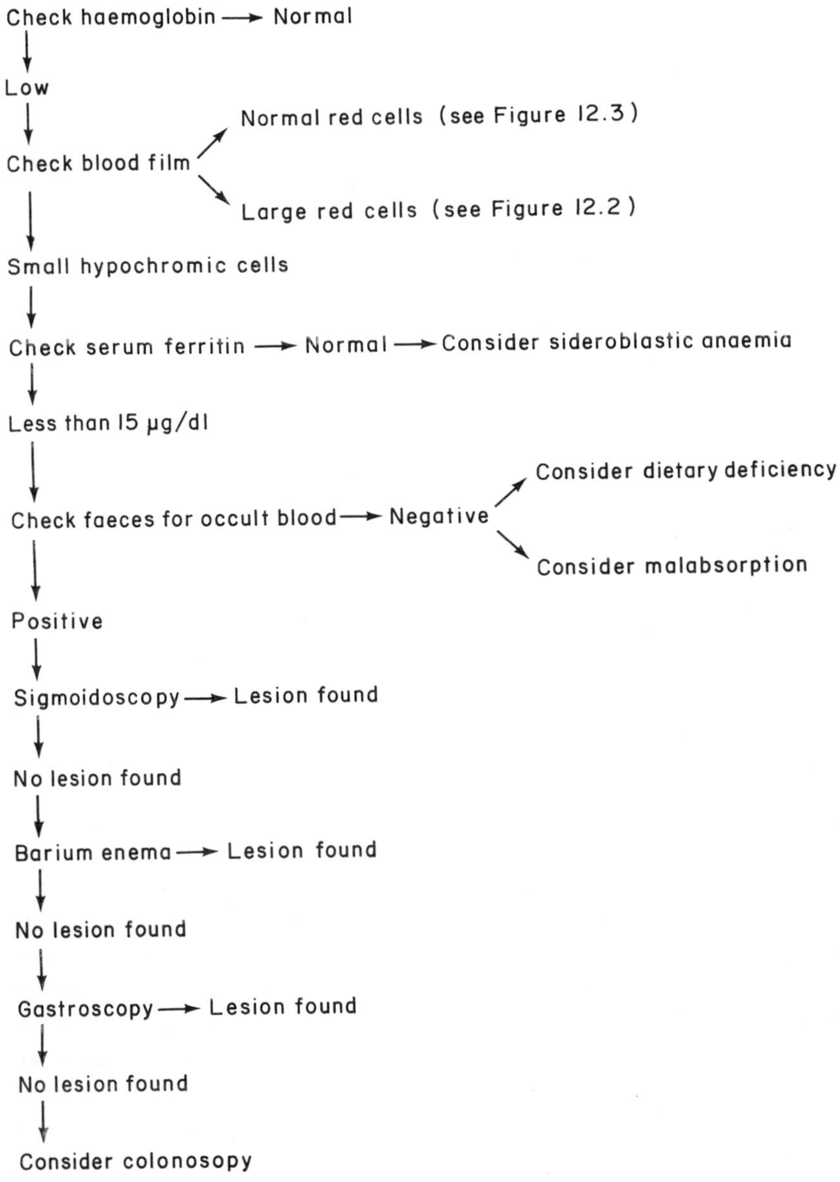

Check haemoglobin ⟶ Normal
↓
Low
↓
Check blood film ⟶ Normal red cells (see Figure 12.3)
⟶ Large red cells (see Figure 12.2)
↓
Small hypochromic cells
↓
Check serum ferritin ⟶ Normal ⟶ Consider sideroblastic anaemia
↓
Less than 15 µg/dl
↓
Check faeces for occult blood ⟶ Negative ⟶ Consider dietary deficiency
⟶ Consider malabsorption
↓
Positive
↓
Sigmoidoscopy ⟶ Lesion found
↓
No lesion found
↓
Barium enema ⟶ Lesion found
↓
No lesion found
↓
Gastroscopy ⟶ Lesion found
↓
No lesion found
↓
Consider colonosopy

Figure 12.1 Laboratory investigation of anaemia. NB. Flow chart assumes that the clinical features were negative. Where these are positive many of the steps may be bypassed

more often a result of gastrointestinal blood loss. The wide range of alimentary lesions that may be responsible for this blood loss have already been described earlier in this chapter. Many pain-relieving tablets may also cause bleeding, the most widely used of which are aspirin, its related compounds and NSAIDs. A considerable amount of persuasion may be necessary to induce patients to stop taking these drugs to which they are often habituated. If they find it difficult to convert to a safer agent such as paracetamol, the NSAIDs can be continued with misoprostol. Steroids may also cause bleeding by increasing acid secretion and inducing peptic ulceration, and this is one of the many reasons for avoiding or minimising their use in the elderly. Unexplained hypochromic ana-

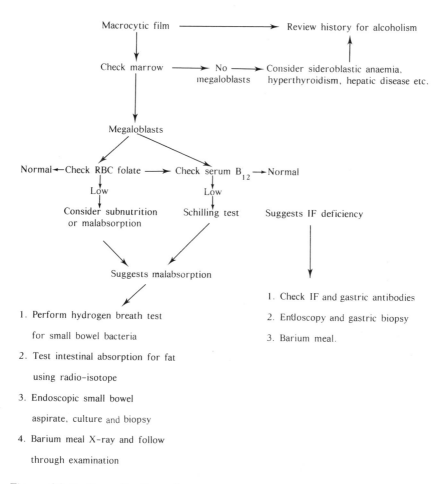

Figure 12.2   Investigation of macrocytic anaemia

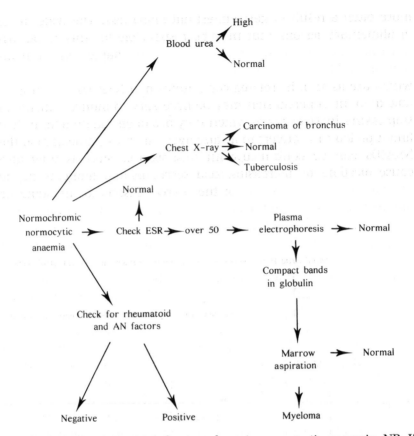

Figure 12.3 Investigation of normochromic normocytic anaemia. NB. If all these investigations are negative, look for evidence of carcinomatosis. Common primary sources are breast, kidney, prostate and thyroid, and sometimes the gut

emia may occasionally be due to gastrointestinal angiodysplasia, which can be very difficult to diagnose in life.

Macrocytic Anaemia

If the blood film contains large red cells (macrocytes) the bone marrow should be aspirated (Figure 12.2), and if microscopic examination shows large red cell precursors (megaloblasts), a diagnosis of vitamin B_{12} or folic acid deficiency is then likely. This can be checked by measuring the blood levels of these two vitamins. B_{12} deficiency may be due to a failure of intrinsic factor (IF) production by the gastric mucosa (due to gastric atrophy), or the overgrowth of B_{12} metabolising bacteria in duodenal or jejunal diverticula, or failure to absorb B_{12} by a diseased terminal ileum, e.g. Crohn's disease. The tests used to differentiate the forms of B_{12} deficiency are shown in Fig. 12.2 (details of the tests will be found in most textbooks of gastroenterology). B_{12} deficiency is treated by injections of cyanocobalamin: a simple regimen is to give 1000 µg on three consecutive days followed by 250 µg at 3-weekly intervals for life.

Folic acid deficiency in old age usually is related to defective nutrition. It rarely is an isolated finding, in that it usually is accompanied by chronic ill health, severe disability or mental impairment. All are situations in which folate intake is liable to be deficient. The red cell folate concentration should be estimated to confirm the diagnosis. Treatment is by folic acid in a dose of 20 mg daily. Serum B_{12} levels should always be checked before folic acid supplements are started because old people are particularly susceptible to the effects of B_{12} depletion which will be accentuated if folic acid is used injudiciously. For example, this could lead to the development of subacute combined degeneration of the spinal cord.

Normochromic Normocytic Anaemia

Many old people suffer from mild anaemia in which the red cells are normal in size (normocytic) and contain normal quantities of haemoglobin (normochromic). It may be due to a wide range of chronic conditions, including rheumatoid arthritis, tuberculosis, renal failure, multiple myeloma and carcinomatosis. Identification of this type of anaemia should lead to a painstaking search for one or more of these disorders (Figure 12.3). Treatment of the anaemia usually involves treatment of the primary condition.

FURTHER READING

Cohen, B. and Thomson, H. (eds) (1986). *Dental Care for the Elderly.* London: Heinemann.

Lawson, D.H. (ed.) (1991). *Current Medicine 3. Royal College of Physicians of Edinburgh.* Edinburgh: Churchill Livingstone.

CHAPTER 13   Metabolic and endocrine aspects

RENAL FUNCTION

Renal blood flow diminishes in a linear fashion with increasing age. The consequences are that reduced renal perfusion causes progressive loss of nephrons and a reduction in the glomerular filtration rate, and changes in the intra-renal blood flow distribution lead to impairment of the distal tubular function. In these circumstances, the older individual is less able to eliminate a water load or alternatively to retain fluid in the face of dehydration. Because the loss of kidney tissue often coincides with a decrease in lean body mass and hence creatinine generation, the serum level of creatinine is not elevated. Conversely, the plasma urea does increase slightly with increasing age but in the absence of pathology does not rise above 10 mmol/1. The consequences of these age-related changes are not apparent in the normal unstressed individual but do mean that there is no or very little renal reserve in the face of stress. Impairment of renal function may be accelerated by a wide range of age-related diseases including hypertension, diabetes, cardiac failure, renal infection and urinary obstruction.

Numerous drugs used in elderly patients rely on the kidneys for their elimination, so that the age-related decrement in renal function must be taken into account when prescribing these drugs and appropriate dosages administered. Table 13.1 lists some of these drugs commonly used in the elderly where dosage reductions are necessary. Many other drugs are also eliminated by the kidneys but in the normal elderly patient, do not require dosage reduction, unless the patient is volume-depleted or has age-related renal pathology.

FLUID BALANCE (Case 2)

The diminution in renal reserve leaves the elderly patient at risk of developing body fluid and body electrolyte imbalance. A minor reduction in cardiac output (cardiac failure) or increased water loss from the lungs during a respiratory infection may induce pre-renal impairment causing a further reduction in the glomerular filtration rate with consequent accumulation of drugs to toxic levels. This is particularly the case with many routinely administered drugs, for example, digoxin (Case 7). Because *total* body water decreases with increasing age, minimal fluid loss causes disproportionate dehydration in elderly patients. The body's osmostat is set at a higher threshold with increasing age so that elderly people are less likely to develop thirst. Equally if they are ill they may be immobilised in bed and inhabit a water desert. Changes in the endocrine control of body fluids leave elderly patients more at risk of developing sodium imbalance—hyper and hyponatraemia.

Table 13.1   Common renal excreted drugs used in elderly patients

---

Antibiotics
Aminoglycosides
Most cephalosporins
Most tetracyclines

Diuretics
Potassium sparing—hyperkalaemia
Thiazides—ineffective
Angiotensin converting enzyme inhibitors—hyperkalaemia

Cardio-active
Digoxin
Disopyramide

Antirheumatics
NSAIDs—fluid retention

Other non-steroidals
Gold
Disodium etidronate

Miscellaneous
Acetolamide
Acyclovir
Baclofen

Reduction in plasma volume elicits an exaggerated response of both antidiuretic hormone (AVP) and atrial natriuretic peptide in older subjects. These responses, and particularly the enhanced AVP response, leave elderly patients at increased risk of developing symptomatic hyponatraemia.

The fluid management of elderly patients is thus very important. Unfortunately, because sick elderly patients are often incontinent, it is difficult to obtain good fluid balance charts. Equally, because of ageing changes in the skin, it is sometimes difficult to make a clinical assessment of hydration. However, monitoring serum electrolytes and body weight represent suitable alternatives to fluid charts (intake and output). Every ward dealing with elderly patients (medical or surgical) should have access to a bed-weighing system so that fluid balance can be monitored. Obviously this is a counsel of perfection and will not be possible in those who are treated at home, and hence may be a reason for requesting admission to hospital.

RENAL AND URINARY TRACT INFECTION (Case 4)

Transient bacteriuria is the norm in otherwise healthy elderly people. In some cases this may be due to inadequate collection techniques though alternatively it may be a consequence of incomplete bladder emptying due to physiological or pathological changes. The collection of mid-stream specimens of urine for microbiological investigation requires a skilled aseptic technique. This particularly applies in the case of elderly women. However, practice (by the nurses!) does make perfect. Rarely is it necessary to resort to the insertion of a catheter or suprapubic aspiration to obtain a clean specimen of urine.

The presence of leucocyturia ($\geq$ 50 cells/ml) indicates infection of the renal tract. In the absence of significant symptoms or declining renal function, there is no consensus as to whether this infection should or should not be treated with antibiotics. Symptoms of lower urinary tract infection (dysuria, frequency, nocturia) or of systemic infection (bacteraemia) should be treated. For presumed community-acquired infections, the antibiotic of choice for a lower urinary tract infection is trimethoprim and for an upper urinary tract infection co-amoxyclav (Augmentin). For hospital-acquired urinary tract infection gentamicin with monitoring of blood levels is to be preferred. For urinary tract infection complicated by bacteraemia, cefotaxime should be used for community-acquired infection and gentamicin combined with ampicillin for hospital-acquired infections. In all cases, specimens (urine and blood) should be sent for culture and sensitivities. In the absence of symptoms of cystitis, urinary tract infection very rarely causes urinary incontinence. Certainly antibiotic treatment of infected urine of an incontinent patient very rarely alters continence (Case 4).

DIABETES MELLITUS

Diabetes mellitus (DM) is the general name for a number of conditions in which there is a failure to control glucose metabolism with consequent hyperglycaemia. The majority of patients fall into one of two groups: Type I insulin dependent (IDDM) and Type II non-insulin dependent (NIDDM). These conditions were previously known as juvenile and maturity onset diabetes respectively but these terms are confusing as both varieties may affect patients across the age range. Diabetes also can be secondary to chronic pancreatitis, drugs (in the elderly thiazide diuretics and corticosteroids are the commonest), hormonal disorders and rarely insulin receptor abnormalities. Both major forms of diabetes, IDDM and NIDDM, give rise to complications of hyperglycaemia manifest by micro- and macrovascular changes. Macrovascular changes are indistinguishable from normal age-related atheromatous change. Macrovascular and other complications—cataract formation, thickening of capillary basement membrane, collagen cross-linking—all occur as age-related phenomena in non-diabetics giving rise to the suggestion that diabetes may be a form of premature or accelerated ageing. Microvascular changes do not, however, occur in healthy persons even in extreme old age.

Aetiology

IDDM is due to an absolute reduction in insulin secretion by the pancreatic islets of Langerhans. Onset is usually but not exclusively before the age of 40 years. There is a genetic and probably an immunological basis for the disease in most patients. Additively or alternatively beta cell damage, directly or indirectly (antigenetic) produced by viral infection, may be a significant factor. The development of NIDDM is very closely associated with obesity and particularly with recent weight gain. Excessive weight gain leads to development of insulin resistance and the pancreatic beta cells are unable to produce sufficient insulin to control hyperglycaemia. Reduction in body weight by dietary means improves glucose tolerance. Ageing by itself also produces a decrease in glucose tolerance. Thus age-related increase in the proportion of body weight which is fat contributes to insulin resistance. A reduction in natural exercise levels with increasing age leads to further impairment of glucose tolerance. Finally the renal threshold for glucose excretion increases with increasing age. Thus the presence of glycosuria in an elderly patient is invariably due to true diabetes (IDDM or more commonly NIDDM) and not just impaired glucose tolerance (Figure 13.1).

Management

The majority of elderly patients with IDDM and a minority with NIDDM present with classical polyuria, polydipsia and weight loss. Polyuria and/or nocturia may be attributed to prostatic hypertrophy (Chapter 14), urinary tract infection, cardiac failure (Chapter 10) or diuretics. Polydipsia and thirst are not so prominent in old age. Often elderly patients present with the complications of diabetes which has been asymptomatic (Table 13.2). A high index of

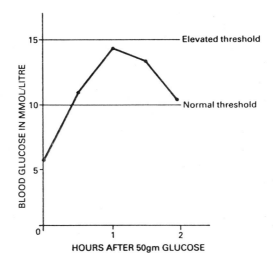

Figure 13.1   Effect of renal threshold of glycosuria in a patient with impaired glucose tolerance

suspicion for the diagnosis is necessary and, if in doubt, the doctor should measure the blood sugar. Fasting levels above 8 mmol/l or post-absorptive ones of more than 11 mmol/l confirm the diagnosis. If doubt still remains an oral glucose (75 g) tolerance test should be performed. The same diagnostic criteria apply to all adults of all ages. Patients should be maintained on an adequate (250 g daily) carbohydrate diet for at least 3 days prior to performing the test.

Specific treatment consists of diet, oral agents or insulin. Diets should be simple and flexible. Advice is best given by a dietitian and the patient's relatives should be present when this is given, if the patient so desires. Restriction of total calorie intake (carbohydrate and fat), in order to reduce weight, should be tried in all patients—occasional success encourages further attempts, but failure should not break the doctor : patient relationship!

The majority of elderly NIDDM patients who do not respond to dietary measures should be treated with short acting sulphonylureas—gliclazide or tolbutamide. Long acting sulphonylureas—glibenclamide and especially chlorpropamide—should no longer be used because of the dangers of hypoglycaemia occurring at night. Any form of recurrent confusion in patients treated with oral agents should be attributed to possible hypoglycaemia until excluded, by measuring blood sugar during the confusional episode (Chapter 9). The confusional state may persist for hours after correction of the blood sugar. Metformin, which is also an appetite suppressant, is useful in obese patients with NNDIM, but occasionally may produce lactic acidosis.

Occasionally, elderly patients may present with IDDM and therefore require insulin treatment. All patients with ketosis or hyperosmolar non-ketotic coma require insulin, at least in the short term. Some patients maintained on diet or oral agents may require short-term insulin treatment to cover acute infection, myocardial infarction, surgery or other form of acute stress. Others may be well controlled with oral agents for many years and then gradually develop increasing hyperglycaemia. There should be no hesitation in switching control to insulin therapy as patients respond with a dramatic increase in well-being.

The management of insulin therapy for many elderly IDDM patients is the same as for younger patients with frequent blood glucose monitoring by the patient. Urinalysis is useless for most elderly due to the high renal threshold for glucose. Patients should attend clinics for glycosylated haemoglobin measurements on a regular basis to monitor overall control. Some may require district nurses to administer injections. However, most can be trained to inject themselves once or twice a day. Here the premixed once daily preparations are very useful.

Complications

Acute ketoacidosis usually occurs in long-standing IDDM patients though sometimes it can be a presenting feature. In the elderly it is usually precipitated by infection, often trivial and overlooked. Less commonly it follows acute myocardial infarction, stroke or trauma (surgical or accidental). Patients are much more likely to present with confusion and impaired consciousness (Chapter 9) than younger subjects, but, otherwise, the signs and symptoms are the same whatever the age of the subject. The only modification of treatment, in the older patient, would be to administer fluid via a central venous pressure (CVP) line to avoid fluid overload and cardiac failure.

Hyperosmolar non-ketotic coma particularly affects elderly patients many of whom were not previously known to be diabetic. The aetiology of the condition is not precisely determined though in some cases it seems to be precipitated by an excess load of carbohydrate often in the form of a "health drink". The hyperosmolality causes rapid loss of consciousness and focal neurological signs are common. Blood glucose levels are often more than 50 mmol/l but pH is normal. Fluid replacement is critical and several litres will need to be given as quickly as possible, via a CVP line, yet avoiding overload and cardiac failure. Insulin should be titrated against blood sugar and electrolyte normality. The dehydration increases plasma viscosity which may cause arterial thromboses which contribute to the high mortality. Recovery of these patients may be slow, with confusion lasting many days after restoration of blood sugar and electrolyte normality.

Other complications

In the main, complications (Table 13.2) of diabetes mellitus, either IDDM or NIDDM, are related to the duration of the disease though the relationship is not very tight. Complications may be apparent when the disease, especially NIDDM, first presents. Alternatively, significant complications may never develop, even when the disease has been treated for 30 years. Microvascular complications seem more related to the disease and its treatment than do macrovascular complications. Similarly there is some evidence that the onset and severity of microvascular changes can be beneficially influenced by tight blood glucose control.

The investigation and management of the ocular, respiratory, renal, cardiac and cerebral complications is the same as in other age groups. However, ocular complications and peripheral vascular disease (PVD) warrant special mention. The treatment of maculopathy and proliferative retinopathy has been revolutionised by the advent of photo- and laser-coagulation techniques. Unfortunately patients will not report visual loss until it is very severe when it is less amenable to treatment. All diabetics, regardless of their age, should have their retinas examined at least yearly. It is mandatory to dilate the pupil to obtain a good view. Older patients should perhaps be examined more frequently, or at least be told to report any visual deterioration as soon as it occurs. Haemorrhages or exudates impinging on the macula or the development of proliferative changes require *immediate* referral to an ophthalmologist if vision is to be preserved.

Good foot care must never be forgotten. The common combination of peripheral neuropathy and arteriopathy (peripheral vascular disease—PVD) causes loss of sensation and relative ischaemia—a dangerous time bomb (Table 13.2). Patients must be

Table 13.2   Complications of diabetes

Vascular	*Ophthalmic*
Cerebrovascular disease	Cataracts
Coronary artery disease	Retinal damage
Peripheral vascular disease	
Postural hypotension	
	Neurological
Infections	Peripheral neuropathy
Pulmonary tuberculosis	Flaccid urinary bladder
Pneumonia	Defective autonomic
Urinary infections	nervous system
Thrush (mouth, vagina, skin)	
Gangrene	
	Renal
Alimentary	Protein leakage
Malabsorption	Chronic renal infection
Diarrhoea	Renal nephropathy

forbidden to attack their feet and toenails with razor blades and other instruments reminiscent of the Inquisition, and told only to use soap and water and then ensure that they dry their feet properly. All other aspects of foot care are the province of the trained chiropodist. Patients should be warned of the dangers and told to seek advice at the earliest stage possible. A minor ingrowing toenail can rapidly progress to local infection and then to extensive necrosis and gangrene requiring above-knee amputation to save life.

THYROID DISEASE

Both overactivity (thyrotoxicosis/hyperthyroidism) and underactivity (myxoedema/hypothyroidism) of the thyroid gland increase with increasing age. The prevalence of hyperthyroidism as shown by screening the elderly is 1% with a M : F ratio of 4 : 1. Hypothyroidism is two to three times commoner with a similar sex ratio. The clinical manifestions of thyroid dysfunction are so protean and/or subtle that routine biochemical screening is probably worthwhile. This is especially the case now that a single test, thyroid-stimulating hormone (TSH) assay can be used to screen for both conditions (Chapter 3).

Hyperthyroidism

Overactivity of the thyroid gland in old age does occur with classical Graves' disease but multinodular goitre and toxic "hot" nodules become commoner in older hyperthyroid patients. Often symptoms of overactivity are classical—increased appetite, sweating, heat intolerance, weight loss, hyperactivity etc. However, a significant minority of patients may present atypically. Thus exophthalmos and the signs of sympathetic overactivity may be less obvious or even absent. Weight loss is usually apparent and may be the only feature. Rarely the condition may be asymptomatic and only be found by coincidental biochemical screening. The heart often bears the brunt of thyroid overactivity in old age and sinus tachycardia, atrial fibrillation and heart failure resistant to usual therapy are common. Rarely the patient may be lethargic, withdrawn and depressed (apathetic thyrotoxicosis of Lahey) so that the doctor has the embarrassment of sending a blood specimen with the query diagnosis of hypothyroidism only to find the results suggest the opposite.

Treatment

Most elderly hyperthroid patients are best treated by a combination of drugs and radioiodine, leaving surgery for the minority with large goitres or nodules and patients who wish for an enhanced cosmetic result. For mild disease, radioiodine should be started first followed a week later by carbimazole. With moderate to severe disease the patient should be made euthyroid with carbimazole before he is given radioiodine. He must be followed up and TSH measured regularly, in the first year at 3 monthly intervals, and thereafter yearly. This programme will identify and treat patients before they develop symptomatic hypothyroidism.

Hypothyroidism

As already mentioned radioiodine treatment of hyperthyroidism causes hypothyroidism. In the past most patients were treated surgically and many of these become hypothyroid. The consequence is that the commonest aetiology for hypothyroidism in the elderly is iatrogenic (post-therapeutic). The next most common cause is autoimmune thyroiditis and more rarely pituitary disorders. The diagnosis is not easy, for many features of the disease are seen in normal ageing (Table 13.3), and therefore needs to be remembered and looked for carefully. The onset and progression of the disease may be so inconspicuous and subtle that the patient's regular medical attendant may miss the diagnosis until a crisis occurs. TSH assays for hypothyroidism therefore should be one of the "screening" tests considered when elderly people "fail to thrive" or are admitted to hospital with non-specific illness (Chapter 3).

The two main complications of hypothyroidism are cognitive impairment and accelerated macrovascular disease (atherosclerosis). The mental symptomatology varies from some minimal mental dullness or slowness through moderate confusion to coma with or without hypothermia (see below). Sadly the cognitive impairment often fails to respond to therapy unless the impairment is very mild. Usually the signs and symptoms are the same as occur in younger adults apart from the hypomania, "myxoedema madness" which rarely occurs in old age.

Table 13.3   Clinical features in ageing and hypothyroidism

Clinical feature	Ageing	Hypothyroidism
Coarse skin	Present	Present
Hair loss	Present	Present
Mental slowness	Often present	Present
Hoarseness	Sometimes present	Present
Reduced sweating	Present	Present
Intolerance to cold	Present	Present
Poor peripheral circulation	Present	Present
Reduced heart rate	Present	Present
Unsteadiness	Usually non-specific	Present (usually)
Constipation	Often present	Present
Poor appetite	Often present	Present

Treatment

Hormone replacement is necessary but the elderly are very sensitive to thyroxine. Invariably hypothyroid patients have considerable coronary atheroma and a sudden increase in metabolic rate may precipitate cardiac failure or myocardial infarction. Therefore the initial dose should be 25 μg once daily. This should be doubled after 2 weeks and again doubled after a further 2 weeks whilst carefully monitoring response and cardiac function. At doses of 100 μg or more, further increase should depend on TSH responses. Many patients are chronically under- or overdosed with thyroxine and maintenance therapy must be determined by the results of TSH measurements (Case 6).

HYPOTHERMIA

Hypothermia is defined as being present when the core temperature of the central body falls below 35 °C. Exposure to cold is the major causative factor. However, hypothermia can occur at the height of an English summer! Social factors such as inadequate heating, poor housing insulation or inappropriate clothing may contribute, but they only produce hypothermia where they are coupled with damage to endogenous temperature regulation. The wide range of factors responsible for this are listed in Table 13.4.

The clinical signs are vague: mild hypothermia may produce pallor, apathy and tachycardia; little else seems amiss. The patient rarely complains of feeling cold. Below 32 °C physical deterioration is more obvious, the signs including a slow irregular pulse, a slow respiratory rate, cold abdomen, muscle rigidity, facial oedema and hypotension; the level of consciousness varies between drowsiness and deep coma.

The essentials for diagnosis include awareness of the possibility and a *low-reading thermometer*. The axillary temperature should be checked and where this is less than 35 °C the rectal temperature should be taken; this differentiates between low skin temperature due to peripheral vasoconstriction and a breakdown in the thermoregulation of the central body core.

Patients with mild hypothermia, if identified and treated, make an uneventful recovery. Mortality is high when the body temperature is less than 32 °C, the death rate exceeding 50%. Complications are related to a disturbance of cardiac function, increased intravascular coagulation and an impaired immunological response to infection (Table 13.5). Systemic and local complications are often silent with minimal symptoms since the body is unable to respond to these pathological conditions. Sadly they become more apparent when the patient warms up.

Table 13.4 Endogenous causes of hypothermia

Brain damage	*Acute illness*
Cerebrovascular disease	Coronary thrombosis
Senile dementia	Pneumonia
Parkinsonism	Pulmonary embolism
	Fractured hip
	Cerebrovascular accident
Suppression of temperature control	
Phenothiazine tranquillisers	*Endocrine disease*
Barbiturates	Hypothyroidism
Tricyclic antidepressants	Adrenal failure
Anticholinergic smooth muscle	Diabetes mellitus
relaxants	
Alcohol	*Increased temperature loss*
	Diminished insulation due to
	loss of body fat
Immobility	Skin disease associated
Neurological disease	with hyperaemia
Osteoarthritis	Large leg ulcers
Rheumatoid arthritis	

Treatment with hot water bottles, an electric blanket or radiant heat are highly effective ways of killing patients with hypothermia because they induce peripheral vasodilatation and the heart is then incapable of maintaining an adequate output for the expanded circulatory system. Hypotension, shock and death are the inevitable consequences.

Reheating must take place very gradually, i.e. $\frac{1}{2}$ °C/hour. In mild cases this can be done by placing the patient in a warm room, and giving him hot drinks. Alcoholic spirits should never be used because they produce vasodilatation which causes further heat loss and a further reduction in core temperature. "Space" blankets stop further heat loss and should be used for all hypothermic patients. In severe cases, with temperatures below 32 °C, admission to hospital and intensive care is essential. Even then treatment should be conservative. There is no evidence that techniques such as heating with a body cradle, mediastinal irrigation, or extracorporeal perfusion produce a lower mortality than gradual rewarming. This should be combined with several ancillary measures: antibiotics are given to prevent or control inevitable chest infection, and dehydration is corrected with appropriate intravenous fluids. Intubation should be avoided since it may provoke ventricular fibrillation and a defibrillator should be available.

Death from hypothermia is best minimised by preventing the condition and old people at risk must be visited regularly, as well as being given advice on clothing, heating and insulation. Disabled people should receive adequate domestic support from either relatives, neighbours or home helps. People with low incomes should be advised of their rights to supplementary heating allowances and supplementary benefits (Chapter 4).

Table 13.5   Complications of hypothermia

Vascular	Alimentary
Mesenteric thrombosis	Pancreatitis
Peripheral gangrene	
Coronary thrombosis	Renal
	Acute renal failure
Respiratory	Cardiac
Pneumonia	Arrhythmia

FURTHER READING

MacLennan, W.J. and Peden, N.R. (1989). *Metabolic and Endocrine Problems in the Elderly*. London: Springer Verlag.

CHAPTER 14 Continence

The importance of social acceptability has already been stressed in Chapter 1. There is no greater cause of embarrassment, stigmatisation and ostracism for patient and carers alike than urinary or faecal incontinence. It is yet another calamity such as blindness, deafness or stroke which often encourages individuals to take a negative view of old age as a period of loss. In order that this should be reversed it is essential that a positive approach should be taken by emphasising the promotion of continence rather than encouraging the attitude that the condition is irreversible and that nothing can be done. National recognition of this was given by founding the British Association for Continence Care (BACC). Over a more prolonged period, research into the condition has been promoted by the International Continence Society (ICS). The essential philosophy is that, until proved otherwise, incontinence should be considered a remediable condition.

URINARY INCONTINENCE (Cases 4 and 8)

Urinary incontinence has been defined as the occurrence of involuntary urinary leakage. Its prevalence varies with the characteristics of the population studied and the precise definition, but in individuals over 65 years living at home, it has been shown to occur regularly in about 12% of women and 7% of men. With increasing age the prevalence increases to about 38% of women and 19% of men over the age of 85 years. This is higher in institutions varying between 40 and 70%, depending on the type of institution.

Urinary incontinence is particularly common in elderly patients admitted to hospital, where it is often due to mental confusion or immobility associated with acute illness, faecal impaction and physical incapacity. The crisis may also be exacerbated by the move to unfamiliar surroundings, and often by inappropriate restriction to bed. In this situation, a patient requesting help with toileting may be told to "wait a minute". Observation has established that the subsequent "minute" may extend to three-quarters of an hour. Intelligent and skilled nursing care minimises the problem, which should resolve once the acute illness is treated and the patient mobilised. In a small proportion of cases the incontinence persists, and requires more detailed assessment.

CAUSES OF PERSISTENT URINARY INCONTINENCE

Neurological Disease

The autonomic nervous system plays an important part in the regulation of bladder function (Figure 14.1). An increase in filling stretches the receptors of afferent fibres. These transmit the information via the spinal cord to efferent fibres, which promote relaxation of the detrusor muscle and relaxation of the urethra with consequent micturition. The process is regulated by fibres from the

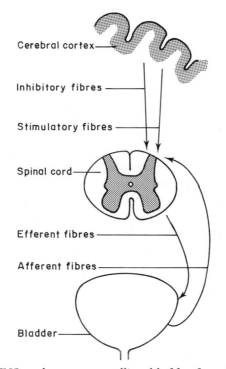

Figure 14.1   CNS pathways controlling bladder function

cerebral cortex which can either enhance the process to produce voluntary micturition, or inhibit it so that the urge is temporarily suppressed. Damage to any part of the system increases the risk of urinary incontinence.

Cerebral cortex

Degenerative and cerebrovascular diseases are the main causes of damage in the elderly. As a result, the suppressant effect on the local spinal cord reflex is reduced so that the bladder has an increased intraluminal pressure, has a reduced volume and empties more frequently.

Spinal cord

Partial destruction of fibres in the spinal cord causes a change in bladder function similar to that due to cortical damage. Complete interruption of the fibres associated with trauma or disorders such as multiple sclerosis is rare in old people and causes a complete loss of control over bladder emptying. Patchy damage due to a poor blood supply, pressure from a prolapsed disc or an early tumour is more common. Incontinence is associated with urgency if sensation is intact. Detrusor muscle contractions (instability) may lead to incontinence without any sensation of the desire to void.

Afferent fibres

Destruction of afferent fibres results in the breakdown of the local bladder reflex arc. Smoooth-muscle fibres then do not contract in response to bladder dilatation, and the bladder fills until it over-flows, so that the patient experiences continuous dribbling incontinence. This may be associated with diabetic neuropathy (Chapter 13).

Local Causes

Local factors are important, often remediable, causes of incontinence. The most common is faecal impaction, where pressure of a loaded rectum on the urethra and bladder interferes with the local reflex and either acute retention or frank urinary incontinence may result. Weakness or damage to the pelvic floor musculature in old women, as a result of neurological disease or as a residuum of childbearing, often leads to an inability to control micturition, and to leakage following sneezing, coughing, laughing or simply a change of posture (stress incontinence). Prostatic enlargement may cause obstruction of the prostatic urethra and retention of urine. This may occur acutely or gradually when it is frequently associated with overflow incontinence and dribbling. In women hypertrophy of the bladder neck may, rarely, give rise to a similar outflow obstruction. Bacteriuria with a count of more than 100 000 organisms per millilitre occurs in about 30% of acute geriatric admissions, and occurs in 6 to 13% of men and 17 to 33% of women living in their own homes. It is unusual for it to cause urinary incontinence unless other symptoms of infection such as frequency and dysuria are present.

Environmental Factors

Incontinence is often accentuated by the interaction between ill health and a hostile environment. Immobility is extremely important. Many old people have difficulty in getting to the lavatory quickly enough. This is particularly important after a cerebrovascular accident where disability, due to hemiparesis, may be accompanied by bladder hyperactivity. Diuretic therapy may also cause incontinence by inducing rapid bladder filling. The design and layout of accommodation and the amount of supporting care available have a direct bearing on the extent to which such factors create problems. Figure 14.2 depicts the continence equation upon which many patients depend for continuing continence.

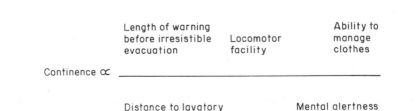

Figure 14.2 The continence equation

MANAGEMENT

If a correct diagnosis is made then treatment can be given and continence restored. The BACC issues a very useful chart which summarises the questions that need to be asked and the steps which need to be taken in order to make a diagnosis and initiate treatment. The basis for an accurate diagnosis rests upon the history of the clinical symptoms and the physical examination.

Symptoms

These will relate to the type of incontinence. There are six main types:

Urge. This occurs in about 85% of men and about 50% of women. The prime symptom is *frequency* combined with **urgency**. The patient passes urine more than six times a day, and has to get up three or more times at night; has to hurry to reach the toilet in time, and has "accidents" if he is unable to achieve this, often wetting the bed at night. The amount of urine passed varies but is often quite small. Passing urine may be painful (dysuria).

Stress. This is uncommon in men but occurs in about 20% of women. The prime symptom is **leaking** small amounts of urine. This happens when the patient coughs, sneezes, strains when lifting things, runs upstairs or makes sudden movements.

Mixed. This is a combination of *urge* and *stress* and is uncommon in the men but occurs in about 30% of the women. The symptoms may be mixed and bladder contractions are triggered by body movements.

Overflow. This occurs in about 10% of men. The prime symptom is "dribbling" in that the stream of urine slows to a dribble and the patient may have to wait for his bladder to empty. Even then it still feels full. The stream is poor, slow to start (hesitancy) and straining may be necessary. Some leaking may occur unconsciously by day or night. Frequency and urgency are also present and, in the early stages of outflow obstruction, the combination of these symptoms with hesitancy, poor stream and dribbling are known as prostatism.

Behavioural. The prime symptom is incontinence for no apparent reason, the patient has no genitourinary symptoms or signs. Urine may be passed without the patient knowing it. Usually the complainant is a relative or carer, and the history one of the patient passing urine in inappropriate places, such as the fireplace, over the banisters or in the umbrella stand.

Nocturnal. A number of patients have nocturnal polyuria which may cause incontinence at night. These patients pass little urine in the day but once they lie down the floodgates open.

Examination

This should be directed particularly towards the central nervous system, the abdomen and genitourinary tract.

Urge incontinence is frequently associated with disorders of the central nervous system, such as cerebrovascular disease, Parkinson's disease, multiple sclerosis or dementia. It may be exacerbated or caused by urinary infection and worsened by psychiatric disorders. A careful examination of the central nervous system should be undertaken as well as assessment of mental state. A specimen of urine should be examined and sent for microscopy and culture.

Stress incontinence is due to laxity of the pelvic floor. It may be associated with utero-vaginal prolapse and atrophic vaginitis, and may occur post prostatectomy in men. Patients should be asked to cough while standing with a half full bladder, when "leakage" will become self-evident.

In *Mixed* incontinence the signs are consistent with both *urge* and *stress* incontinence.

Overflow incontinence is commonly due to obstruction to the flow of urine resulting from prostatic enlargement in men or a bladder neck obstruction in women due to a pelvic mass, such as fibroids or uterine prolapse. Faecal impaction may also be a cause in both sexes. Physical signs include evidence of a poor stream and dribbling on micturition, a palpable bladder, evidence of uterine prolapse, or a pelvic mass on vaginal examination. Rectal examination may confirm impaction or an overloaded bowel may be felt on abdominal palpation. Since faecal impaction is frequently associated with neurological disease, such as stroke, Parkinson's disease and spinal injury, examination of the nervous system must be made. Drugs with an anticholinergic action may also contribute to *overflow*.

Behavioural incontinence may be associated with signs of mental impairment or disorientation. Alternatively no abnormal physical signs may found. In these cases, as in all cases of incontinence the completion of a frequency/volume incontinence chart (Figure 14.3) may be invaluable and indicate a possible cause. Random incontinence may be due to disorientation in strange surroundings

INCONTINENCE CHART

Surname: Hesketh

Christian Name: Gloria

Unit No: SE 279051

Ward: Marlborough

Date of Admission: 13. 3. 93   **Time:** 2145 hrs

Date:	14. 3. 93		15. 3. 93		16. 3. 93	
Time	Toilet or bed pan Given by	U.F. or dry (Amount)	Toilet or bed pan Given by	U.F. or dry (Amount)	Toilet or bed pan Given by	U.F. or dry (Amount)
0200	A/N White	U ?100mls				
0400	A/N Scott	U ?50mls				
0600	A/N Scott Bed Pan	D 80mls				
0800	A/N Hart Toilet	D 100mls				
1000	A/N Hart Toilet	D Nil				
1200	R.N Lane Toilet	U ?100mls				
1400	SEN John Toilet	D 120mls				
1600	SEN John Toilet	D 150mls				
1800	SEN John Toilet	D 120mls				
2000	S/N Evans Toilet	D 70mls				
2200	A/N White Toilet	D 100mls				
2400	A/N White	U ?50mls				

Figure 14.3 A form of incontinence chart with an example of information recorded over 24 hours

or be a silent protest indicating distress or dissatisfaction with their present social situation.

Nocturnal incontinence may sometimes be due to low grade chronic heart failure.

Special Investigations

If possible, a "clean catch", mid-stream specimen of urine should be examined microscopically for cytology and cultured for bacterial contamination. Further investigation is dependent on the findings of the history and physical examination. In many cases the diagnosis is clear and treatment can be started (Figure 14.4). In others,

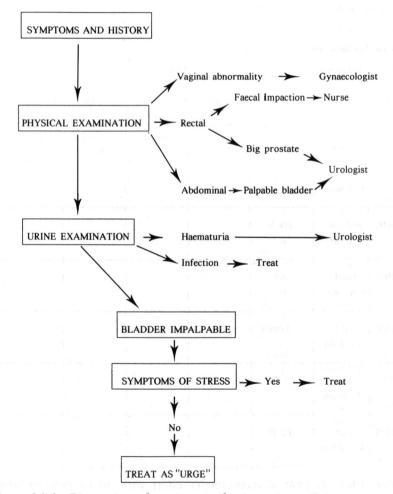

Figure 14.4 Diagnosis and treatment of urinary incontinence

referral to a specialist (urologist, geriatrician or gynaecologist) may be indicated and further specialist investigation may be necessary if the diagnosis remains in doubt. In many centres geriatricians, urologists and gynaecologists collaborate closely, and urodynamic studies are undertaken by all.

Overflow incontinence in men is commonly the late stage of outflow obstruction due to prostatic enlargement, and should have been treated before this stage is reached. The simplest way of making the diagnosis is to measure the residual urine, after voiding, by in/out catheterisation. However, this is an invasive procedure and some practitioners prefer to get the patient to complete a frequency/volume chart over a period of a week, measure his urinary flow rate, and post-micturition residual urine using ultrasound. Since surgery will be necessary, routine investigations are needed and should include haemoglobin and full blood count, plasma urea and electrolytes, serum acid phosphatase or prostate-specific antigen. If the prostate feels hard or irregular on rectal examination, a needle biopsy should be taken under rectal ultrasound control, to exclude cancer, and stage the disease, if present.

Treatment

This should be directed at eliminating the cause, or, if this is not possible, at preventing or minimising the problem.

Urge incontinence is best treated by bladder retraining. The aim of this is to reduce bladder irritability by increasing its capacity. Patients need to keep a micturition record and gradually try to increase the period between voiding. This has the effect of stretching the bladder and reducing instability. Any urinary infection should be treated with an appropriate antibiotic. The aim of a toileting regime is to achieve dryness by getting the patient to void before the sensation of a desire to void arises. If he waits for the sensation of urgency he may have waited too long because when he stands up the detrusor contracts and he leaks. Advice should be given with regard to fluid intake, avoidance of alcohol and caffeine containing liquids, diuretic therapy unless unavoidable, and attention to bowel function. The lavatory must be easily accessible. Drugs with an anticholinergic action such as oxybutynin 2.5 to 5 mg two to four times daily may help to reduce detrusor instability and increase bladder capacity. The district continence adviser and support nurses are indispensable in providing support and advice to the patient, carer and primary care team. Bedwetting at night can be extremely distressing to these patients and their carers. This can be prevented by voiding at regular intervals during the night. Avoiding hypnotics and arranging an alarm call (or a series of alarm calls) may also be required to establish a pattern that prevents enuresis.

Stress incontinence may respond to simple measures unless pelvic floor weakness is severe. Weight reduction in the obese, prevention of constipation, removal of tight corsets and exercises to strengthen the pelvic floor muscles may be successful in mild cases. Pelvic muscle tone can be successfully increased in younger women by teaching them to insert serial weight cones into the vagina. This, however, needs a high degree of motivation and cooperation and may be of less use in the older patient. Local oestrogens counteract atrophic changes and may produce improvement (Case 8). Pessaries, rings or tampons may also be used in those cases that do not respond to simple measures. Their use should be considered as a temporary measure pending surgical reconstruction, unless the patient is unfit for surgery.

Overflow incontinence, if due to outflow obstruction, almost always requires surgical intervention, unless it is due to faecal impaction in which case disimpaction will produce a cure. When the cause is an atonic bladder some patients are able to empty their bladders either by manual expression or triggering a reflex response by some action which is individual to them, e.g. repetitively stroking the inner aspect of the thigh. If this is unsuccessful it may be possible to teach some patients intermittent self-catheterisation but if this fails an indwelling catheter may be needed as a last resort.

Other types of incontinence often respond to treatment if the cause can be determined. When it is associated with mild intellectual impairment, perhaps a symptom of early dementia (Chapter 9), it may respond to a toileting programme combined with reality orientation. Sometimes the incontinence follows a move and settles as the individual gets used to the new surroundings. Rarely it may be wilful, as an attempt to manipulate a situation. If this is the case, the reason should be sought, remedied if possible, and the patient and, perhaps, carer(s) counselled.

Benign Prostatic Hypertrophy

Transurethral resection of the prostate (TURP) is the commonest procedure performed to relieve the obstruction caused by this condition. Most patients are fit for this and the operative mortality is approximately 1 to 2%. The operation may be done under spinal or general anaesthesia. American experience suggests that about a third of men over 40 years will eventually require a prostatectomy but though about three-quarters of men over 50 years suffer from symptoms suggesting an enlarged prostate, most will not require surgery. If all patients with symptoms were to require operation the economic implications would be enormous. It is not surprising, therefore, that other methods of treatment are being sought. These include balloon dilatation, urethral stents, hyperthermia and drugs. Drugs which show the greatest promise are those directed at influencing muscular tone in the prostatic capsule and bladder neck, such as alpha-adrenoceptor antagonists, or agents which prevent prostatic growth by blocking the conversion of testosterone to dihydro-testosterone by inhibiting 5-alpha-reductase. However, the symptoms of benign prostatic hypertrophy fluctuate considerably and new treatments must undergo rigorous appraisal before their value can be recommended.

Prostatic Cancer

Treatment depends on the staging of the disease. Transrectal ultrasound is helpful in this respect for it will not only allow accurate needle biopsy but indicate the degree of local spread. If the disease is confined to the prostate and bone scans have shown no metastatic spread, TURP alone is probably sufficient. If the disease has spread locally, has metastasised or is poorly differentiated then anti-androgen therapy will be necessary as well. The simplest and most cost-effective treatment is orchidectomy, though some authorities believe that all patients with prostatic cancer should receive long-term treatment with goserelin (Zoladex) monthly implants. Cyproterone acetate may be given as second line treatment to those patients who do not respond.

Haematuria

This is common in the elderly, more so in men than women. A very small quantity of blood in the urine gives an appearance of redness out of proportion to the actual quantity lost. Painless haematuria is commonly a symptom of bladder cancer, while painful haematuria is usually associated with infection (Figure 14.4). In both cases the patient should be referred to a urologist for further investigation to exclude malignancy. All patients should have ultrasonography and an intravenous pyelogram to exclude renal carcinoma (hypernephroma) and bladder tumour.

INCONTINENCE AIDS

When incontinence cannot be controlled, steps should be taken to minimise its effects and the embarrassment it causes. However, as a first step, the incontinence must be reviewed to ensure that a correct diagnosis has been made and that no remediable condition has been missed. The incontinence chart (Figure 14.3) should be monitored, to check the frequency and volume of urine loss. Solutions relating to the adjustment of the environment, ability to manage clothing, and the provision of a commode should all be considered. A decision has to be made as to whether the patient can be managed with pads alone, a condom attached to a urinal (in men) or a permanent indwelling catheter, with or without attachment to a urinal. The local continence advisory service can be a great help in reaching the most effective decision, in consultation with the patient and the carer.

Urinals

Portable urinals may be very helpful in the management of "urge" incontinence in that they enable patients to be able to micturate easily and cleanly with a minimal degree of embarrassment. All urinals should have a non-returnable valve. The Femisep or similar slim urinals are useful for female patients and the Reddy-Bottle, which has a one-way valve and is disposable, is useful when travelling. When incontinence cannot be controlled males can be fitted with a condom which connects via a tube to a leg bag. At night a similar apparatus, with a non-return valve, may be used. Mental capacity and manual dexterity are of major importance to a patient adapting to such a device, and a considerable amount of training by both nurse and occupational therapist may be necessary before the individual becomes proficient.

Incontinence Pads

No practical urinal has yet been developed for the incontinent female, and resort has to be made to water-absorbent materials. A small discrete absorbent pad can be used for stress incontinence. Larger shaped pads containing a super absorbent material combined with a deodorant are used to accommodate heavier urinary leakage. These are kept in place with net pants or fitted into a marsupial pouch in special designed pants.

At night when the patient is in bed, the mattress should be protected. The simplest form of protection is the well-known pad, comprising a sheet of water-absorbent paper with a waterproof backing. The disadvantage of this is that the patient has to lie on a damp surface, and will be at risk of developing bed sores (Chapter 5). A better solution is to cover the mattress with a plastic sheet and use a reusable underpad (e.g. Kylie) "one-way" material which allows urine to drain through but retains a dry surface in contact with the skin.

Catheterisation

Short-term catheterisation should be used to control incontinence where there is urinary retention, sacral pressures sores (Chapter 5) or other open wounds, or when the patient is unconscious. Teflon encapsulated catheters can be used for up to 28 days. When all else fails, long-term catheterisation has to be considered. This may be the only way of keeping the patient dry, or of healing macerated skin. It is doubtful if this measure should ever be used to reduce laundry expenses or nursing workload.

When the patient has to be catheterised infection can be minimised by using a meticulous aseptic technique. The choice of catheters is between hydrogel "Biocath" or an all silicone catheter. Rubber or uncoated catheters are toxic and should no longer be used. Urine should be allowed to drain freely into a non-returnable leg bag, or into a bag attached around the waist (Shepherd's sporran). Intermittent catheter drainage, by causing bladder stasis, is invariably followed by infection. It should be avoided when catheterisation is permanent but may be useful when it is intended to withdraw the catheter and restore continence (as in postoperative retention of urine in women). Four-hourly emptying prevents the bladder from becoming small and hypertonic. Bladder washouts are of little value in preventing infection and are best avoided as a routine measure.

Leakage around the catheter can sometimes be a problem particularly in women. The Bard Conforma catheter overcomes this problem and is more comfortable to wear. Conversely, leakage is likely to be less if a smaller catheter (12–16 Ch) with a small balloon (5–10 ml) is used rather than a large one. Bladder relaxants, such as oxybutinin, may also be useful. Catheters should be changed as infrequently as possible, and ideally should last up to 3 months.

FAECAL INCONTINENCE

Faecal incontinence is much less common than loss of bladder control. Table 14.1 lists causes in the elderly, the most important of these being faecal impaction.

Faecal Impaction (Case 3)

Faecal impaction is caused by a combination of slow transit in the colon, lack of physical exercise and patients neglecting the call to stool, as happens in the disabled who have difficulty in getting to the lavatory. Finally, sheer physical weakness may make faecal evacuation difficult. The faeces in people with faecal impaction tend

Table 14.1 Causes of faecal incontinence

Faecal impaction
Diarrhoea due to:
  dietary indiscretion
  bacterial or viral infection
  purgative abuse
  diverticular disease
  cancer
Leakage of liquid paraffin
Pelvic floor damage with:
  lax anal sphincter
  rectal prolapse
Loss of colonic inhibition due to:
  dementia
  cord damage

to be soft rather than "rock hard" and the traditional picture of a hard lump of faeces with liquid faeces above is probably only present in about 10% of faecally incontinent elderly patients.

Faecal incontinence due to faecal impaction may present as the leakage of liquid faeces from the anus, when fluid material in the more proximal part of the colon bypasses the impaction lower down. The fluid has a distinctive and foul odour, and may sometimes be mistaken for "diarrhoea". The diagnosis is made by identifying large amounts of soft faeces in the rectum and lower colon. Digital examination of the rectum is usually sufficient to make the diagnosis, but occasionally high faecal impaction is associated with an empty rectum. In these cases a plain abdominal X-ray can be helpful in making the diagnosis.

Treatment

The condition can usually be treated by giving an enema, and repeating this until the colon is radiologically empty. Soap and water enemas should never be used, for they cause disastrous dehydration and haemoconcentration; small hypertonic phosphate enemas (micro-enemas) are equally effective and are virtually free from side effects.

Once the colon has been emptied of faeces, regular bowel actions must be maintained. Traditionally, in hospital this task is often left to the nursing staff, and, while it is right for nurses to continue to supervise bowel function, accurate records must be kept and bowel control reviewed regularly on ward rounds, case conferences or home visits, so that appropriate regimes are prescribed by the doctor and the patient trained in their use, and constipation prevented in the future.

Constipation

A wide range of laxatives is available but relatively few are of value in old age.

Bran. Bran added to the food is a very effective way of increasing colonic roughage content, as is the consumption of fruit, fresh vegetables and fibrous cereals. But bran should only be given when the faeces are hard. If the faeces are soft, bran will only increase colonic content and worsen faecal soiling and incontinence.

Lactulose. Faecal bulk can be increased by using lactulose. Fermentation of this synthetic disaccharide in the colon produces frequent soft stools. It also produces gas which often gives rise to flatulence, and abdominal discomfort. The dose should be related to the response (Chapter 5).

Stool softeners and lubricants. Old people find it difficult to pass hard faeces and stool softening agents can be of value in this situation. Liquid paraffin was used for many years but if aspirated can cause pneumonia and when taken in excess or incorrectly will cause anal leakage. It has no place in present day treatment.

Stimulant laxatives. Drugs with a local irritant effect on the colon seem to be reasonably effective as laxatives. Standardised senna in a dose of one or two tablets daily is a suitable preparation, although some patients prefer equivalent doses of senna in the form of granules or a syrup. Bisacodyl in a dose of one or two tablets is a useful alternative. More powerful irritants such as castor oil are of historical interest; they have no place in present day therapy.

Dioctyl sodium sulphosuccinate is an effective stimulant and softening agent with few proven side effects. Concern has been expressed about its possible long-term effects on gastrointestinal absorption, but these are of theoretical rather than practical significance. Dosage is 200 mg three times a day initially, reducing to 200 mg on alternate days.

Advice on how to prevent impaction must be given to the patient once the episode has been dealt with. He should visit the lavatory once a day and attempt to pass faeces even though he has had no call to stool. Easy access to the lavatory must be ensured so that he can comply with this requisite. This may involve altering the house, fitting appropriate rails, building an indoor lavatory, or even moving to more satisfactory accommodation. However, the provision of a commode may be a simpler solution!

Patients must be warned emphatically about the dangers of laxative overdosage. Examples including severe potassium depletion or defective gut innervation (melanosis coli) resulting from this habit are by no means rare in geriatric practice, and the need to pass motions daily should not be overstressed. Finally, improving general health and mobility is an essential element in preventing a recurrence of faecal impaction, for the condition is predominately a disorder of the sick and the chairbound.

Diarrhoea (Case 4)

Old people are frequently incontinent of faeces when they suffer an attack of diarrhoea; they are "taken short" unable to get to the lavatory in time. Symptomatic treatment with anti-diarrhoeal drugs usually alleviates the condition and the patient's distress. The disorder must be taken seriously and if there is not an immediate response to treatment further investigation should be undertaken. Patients with severe diarrhoea or who are incontinent with diarrhoea may have sinister underlying bowel disease. Dehydration and electrolyte disturbance can occur rapidly and admission to hospital for treatment and fluid replacement may be necessary. It should also be remembered that the elderly may travel far and wide, so that dysentery, both amoebic and bacillary, is not uncommon. If the stool is too soft there is an increased risk of leakage and this can be treated with a constipating drug such as loperamide or codeine.

Mental Impairment

A few patients with dementia may simply defaecate in inappropriate places. This usually occurs when brain disease has reached an advanced stage, and the patient has developed faecal loading or impaction. Twice weekly enemas, micro- rather than saline, usually control the problem. Occasionally a constipating regime (loperamide or codeine) with weekly enemas is required.

FURTHER READING

Brocklehurst, J.C. (1984). *Urology in the Elderly*. Edinburgh: Churchill Livingstone.

Castleden, C.M. and Duffin, H. (1991). *Staying Dry: Advice for Sufferers of Incontinence*. Lancaster: Quay Publishing.

Mandelstram, D. (1986). *Incontinence and its Management*, 2nd Edn. London: Chapman & Hall.

Mares, P. (1990). *In Control. Help with Incontinence.* London: Age Concern (England).

Smith, M. and Clamp, M. (1991). *Continence Promotion in General Practice* (Practice Guides for General Practice 13). Oxford: Oxford University Press.

CHAPTER 15   Terminal care

In the last edition of this book it was stated that the death rate in most geriatric units was 30% of all admissions, and it was thought that since the proportion of the very old in the population would increase, this figure was likely to rise. In fact, a recent study suggests that although there has been a rise in the number of hospital admissions, there has been an increase in the number of discharges from hospital of people who were in the last year of their lives. Moreover, comparatively few of those aged 85 years or more died in hospital compared with their younger peers. This is probably due to the considerable increase in the number of residential/nursing homes. It has also been suggested that cancer in old people is often badly treated, unless they are admitted to a hospice. This is unlikely, since the number of hospice places being limited are taken up by younger age groups. It would seem, therefore, that the trend is for many older people to die outside the hospital setting and that all doctors, nurses, social workers and carers looking after the elderly should study the problems of pain, death and bereavement.

THE MANAGEMENT OF THE DYING

The treatment of the dying patient raises many ethical issues, a clinician's approach to these being governed by his cultural background and general attitude to life. Dogmatic pronouncements are inappropriate to this aspect of medical and nursing care, but despite this, considerable training, experience, skill and judgement is involved in the management of terminal illness and the handling of bereaved relatives. An increasing proportion of doctors, nurses and social workers have developed an interest in this difficult field, and their writings have provided us with many useful and practical guidelines.

To Treat or Not to Treat? (Cases 9 and 10)

A doctor is sometimes faced with the question of whether a particular illness should be treated, for treatment may not prolong worthwhile life, but only produce a more lingering and uncomfortable death. The problem rests with the definition of "worthwhile" and who makes the definition. The difficulty is that decisions often have to be taken with inadequate information. For example, the elderly patient with delirium (Chapter 9) may also have dementia and have been a burden to carers, society and himself for some time: on the other hand his condition may be due to an acute respiratory infection superimposed on previously undiagnosed lung cancer. In both cases the question of appropriate treatment arises, and, in making a decision, as much information as possible should be obtained about the past history from relatives, neighbours, the general practitioner, district nurses, health visitor, social workers, other carers and any other person who knows the individual well. Enquiry should also try to establish whether the patient has any known preferences. At the present time debate is taking place on the topic of the "Living Will", and some people have expressed their wishes in writing. While this does not have the legal weight in the UK that it does in Holland, it may be a useful guide to the doctor.

The choice is rarely between treatment and no treatment. In most cases the patient is capable of expressing his own opinion, and it is only when this is impossible that difficult decisions may be needed. Even then, when a decision has been taken not to prevent death, active measures must be taken to prevent suffering, and doctors will need to use all their skill to achieve this. Thus treatment may be necessary to relieve breathlessness (Case 9) in terminal pneumonia, to control obstruction of the vena cava in lung cancer or to relieve the pain of bony secondaries. Such steps may involve doctors from different disciplines in the management of the patient, and may involve them in apparently complex measures. These may be entirely justified if they enable the patient to die with dignity and in comfort.

What to Tell the Patient (Case 9)

A great deal of attention has been given to the question of whether or not the patient should be told that he is dying. This depends to some extent on the patient and the diagnosis. If the condition is associated with gross intellectual impairment, discussion with the patient is obviously futile. Again, in acute illness, of whatever nature, accurate prediction of outcome is impossible even when death is probable. Even when the patient has cancer, prognostication can be difficult, for progression of the tumour may be extremely variable in old age. Many people with breast or other cancers live for years after the diagnosis has been made, and often die from causes unrelated to their cancer. It is likely also that many patients already know they have cancer, for age is no bar to aggressive treatment of disease and this should have been discussed with them.

Despite these exceptions, there remains a small group of alert patients in whom the outcome is clear, even though the time span is difficult to predict. The least exacting approach is for the relatives and supporting staff to maintain a facade of false optimism, but this is rarely effective and they are ultimately forced into inventing a whole web of fabrication. Once the patient detects the deception he loses faith with all concerned, and his behaviour alters: he may simply give up asking questions and withdraw into apathy. More usually, to avoid embarrassment, he plays everyone else's game pretending to believe in a favourable prognosis. Often this will place barriers between the patient, the professional carers and relatives so that the eventual crisis is faced alone and unsupported.

Unvarnished frankness may also lead to considerable distress. Pronouncement of a death sentence may be followed by a period of disbelief and denial. When the truth becomes apparent the patient may struggle against the inevitable by going from doctor to doctor, by attempting to bargain for life with a deity, or by altering life-long habits which are thought to relate to the illness. When this fails an alternative target to the predicament is sought which, all too frequently, is the "nearest and dearest", thereby undermining life-long love and regard; nursing and medical staff may also become involved. Escape may also take the form of depression and complete withdrawal.

Supporting staff can avoid this sequence of events by understanding the patient, the family and their dilemma. The essential starting point is to get to know the patient. He has the right to confidentiality and, however anxious the family, no discussion of the illness should be undertaken without first obtaining the patient's permission. Usually this presents no problem, for patients will ask the direct question "What is wrong with me?", and in answering this one can enquire if the patient wants others told;

when he does not, the question should be asked when the initial history is taken, and recorded in the notes. This is frequently forgotten, unless it is something which is done routinely. Once the answer to this question (Do you want your spouse/next of kin to be told about your illness?) is known, then it is easy to ask the next question, "Do you want to know the details of what is wrong with you?" (Case 9).

Fortunately most patients are quite happy for their medical problems to be discussed with their spouse or next of kin, but it is wise to make sure that this is so. Whether that information is given to others can then be left to the patient and those he wishes to be informed. All patients are different in their attitudes and while some will want to know all the details, particularly with regard to the eventual outcome, so that they can make appropriate plans, others will not want to know and will accept explanations even though suspecting the worst. Direct lies should always be avoided. The hope of the patient for a normal, comfortable life and that of the family for improvement should always be maintained, however unlikely this may seem.

The amount of time spent in maintaining morale is never wasted. The length of discussion varies. In a few instances it may be possible to make a complete exposition within a few sentences, but it is rare for patients to "take in" what the doctor has said without repetition. "They never tell you anything" is a common remark for patients, and their relatives, to make after a detailed doctor : patient consultation. Planned "informal" chats with the patient, and the relatives if he agrees, are a good way of helping better understanding. The "out of hours" visit to the hospital bedside or patient's home may be necessary. This is time consuming but well worthwhile and usually greatly appreciated.

Terminal care is a team event, whether it takes place in hospital or at home. Many health care professionals and others will be involved. Unless the patient is already well known to members of the team, details of his personality, relationship with his family, strengths and weaknesses, fears and anxieties only emerge over a period of days or weeks. It is essential that the team pool information and that the information the patient gleans from different members of the team does not contain major discrepancies. Detailed notes of all important conversations with the patient and between members of the team are absolutely essential to achieve this; these should be kept in the case records to which all members of staff have access and to which they should contribute. A separate sheet of a distinguishing colour may prove a useful addition to the notes. All team members can then summarise on this any communication with the patient and relatives.

Relief of Symptoms (Cases 9 and 10)

Sympathetic discussion is of little avail if the patient remains uncomfortable and distressed. Doctors looking after dying patients must be skilled in the use of drugs, particularly those which relieve pain and modify mood, the objective being to keep the patient comfortable and alert.

Relatively mild analgesics are often successful in controlling pain if they are taken regularly; they are less effective if taken only when the pain recurs, and in this situation the patient comes to dread the return of pain. Whenever possible patients should be trained to control their own medication for the relief of their pain and record the time and amount of each dose. Anxiety, coupled with a psychological adaption to the drug used, results in the acquisition of tolerance and the need for larger and larger doses. The doctor is then faced with the choice of making the patient unconscious or leaving him in pain. Regular dosage at adequate levels should minimise both anxiety and drug tolerance. The fact that an agent is a narcotic should not be a barrier to its administration. Even heroin (diamorphine) given for several months does not produce addiction in terminal illness so long as the doses are given regularly and kept at the minimum necessary for effective relief of pain.

Table 15.1 lists some of the drugs of value in the relief of pain. Morphine and diamorphine remain the most potent analgesics. Sustained release morphine (MST Continus) tablets may be useful in reducing the number of doses required, while intravenous infusions of morphine given by a pump may provide excellent relief (Case 10). Long acting and intravenous morphine also allows the patient to sleep through the night without being wakened for a repeat dose of morphine. Sleep may help to raise the pain threshold, and hypnotics with a short duration of action, so that oversedation is avoided, can be useful in the early stages of treatment. Examples are the short acting benzodiazepines (temazepam, lormetazepam) and chlormethiazole. Sleeplessness may also be a symptom of depression (Chapter 9) and lofepramine given at night will improve insomnia obviating the need for an hypnotic. Aspirin and other NSAIDs may be very useful in relieving bone pain produced by bony secondaries. Steroids may also be helpful in producing euphoria or a sense of well-being as well as reducing hypercalcaemia associated with bone secondaries from a primary carcinoma of breast or lung.

Pain is often associated with anxiety. Sympathy and explanation will help to relieve this, but anxiolytics may also be needed. (Table 15.2 lists some suitable agents.) Local radiotherapy is especially useful for painful metastases.

Attention should be directed to other distressing symptoms. Breathlessness (Case 9) should be dealt with by treating the cause. If, following this, the condition persists or is associated with a painful cough, suppression of respiration with a narcotic preparation such as methadone linctus should be considered. Morphine has also been shown to be of value in relieving respiratory distress in motor neurone disease.

Vomiting is a distressing feature of many terminal illnesses and may complicate therapy. Table 15.3 lists some useful anti-emetic agents. Hyoscine, although an anti-emetic, causes restlessness and confusion in old people and should not be used. If the symptom is due to gastrointestinal obstruction palliative surgery should always be considered, the discomfort of an operation having to be balanced against the distress of persistent vomiting and starvation. Metabolic causes such as hypercalcaemia must also be remembered.

Terminal illness is often associated with gross wasting due to a combination of increased protein breakdown and poor nutrient intake. It is usually followed by the onset of pressure sores, unless extreme care is taken of pressure points and preventive aids used, such as alternating pressure mattresses (Chapter 5). Anabolic drugs, such as the oral agent stanozolol, merit consideration; they not only reduce weight loss, but have a mild euphoriant effect. Tissue breakdown can be delayed further by the administration of ascorbic acid or zinc. Care of the terminally ill elderly patient is often difficult in an acute ward, and setting up a palliative care ward within the geriatric unit has been shown to be of value, a 12 bed ward caring for up to 128 patients in the year. Such a ward has an obvious role in clinical research, teaching and training, as well as benefiting patients and their relatives. It also means that staff can concentrate on a single issue and are not sidetracked by heterogeneous problems; nurses become skilled in counselling, while other specialists with skills in pain control, oncology and radiotherapy can advise as necessary.

Table 15.1 Analgesics

Drug	Analgesic effect	Anxiolytic effect	Dose	Route	Side effects
Aspirin	+	−	600 mg	Oral	−
Paracetamol	+	−	0.5–1 g	Oral	−
Co-proxamol	++	+	2 tablets	Oral	
Codeine	+	−	30 mg	Oral	Constipation
Dihydrocodeine	++	−	30–60 mg	Oral	Constipation
Methadone linctus	++	−	5–10 mg	Oral	−
Morphine	+++	+++	8–20 mg	Subcutaneous	Vomiting, constipation
Diamorphine	+++	+++	5–10 mg	Intramuscular	Vomiting, constipation
MST Continus	+++	+++	10–60 mg	Oral	Vomiting, constipation

Note: Only side effects likely to be of importance in terminal illness are recorded.

Table 15.2   Oral anxiolytics

Drug	Daily dosage
Chlorpromazine	25–50 mg
Thioridazine	10–50 mg
Promazine	50 mg
Diazepam	2–20 mg
Chlordiazepoxide	5–40 mg

Table 15.3   Oral anti-emetics

Drug	Sedative effect	Dose
Cyclizine	++	25–50 mg
Metoclopramide	–	5–10 mg
Domperidone	–	10–30 mg
Promazine	+	25–75 mg
Chlorpromazine	+	10–25 mg
Ondansetron	–	8–16 mg

Note: None of these drugs has side effects that are likely to be of importance in terminal illness.

BEREAVEMENT

Bereavement is usually associated with with a sense of loss and of loneliness which may go on to produce a true depression (Chapter 9). Paradoxically, a sense of relief is often felt when death occurs and this may be followed by a distressing sense of guilt. This is especially common when illness has been prolonged or when hospital admission immediately precedes death. The stress of bereavement may also cause very real illness. There is an increased death rate in spouses and siblings in the first year of bereavement.

These hazards can be reduced by careful counselling before and after death. Grief is a healthy reaction and should be encouraged. Evidence exists that sharing grief with the dying person reduces the effect of grief after bereavement; the fact that close relatives have been able to discuss the subject with the patient and been able to comfort one another acts as a balm to both parties. Total suppression of grief may result in its effects being even more distressing later on.

In the period immediately following death, treatment should consist of providing sympathy and giving advice about adjusting to changed circumstances. Hypnotics may be useful for a short time to re-establish sleep pattern. Relatives and friends should be counselled to maintain contacts. Loneliness is frequently induced because the widow(er) is left to mourn alone, because neighbours and friends are embarrassed to "intrude on his grief", or are rebuffed by the bereaved who gives the impression that "he wants to be left alone with his grief". Counteracting such misapprehensions needs tact and time. If after several weeks he remains severely distressed the possibility of depression must be considered; this often responds well to antidepressant drugs.

MALIGNANCY

The incidence of most malignant conditions rises with increasing age. Details of some of these have already been dealt with in the appropriate section and it is only the intention here to make some general comments and briefly discuss some common cancers which have not yet been mentioned.

Malignancy in the elderly differs from that in the rest of the population in several important respects.

1. Because of their limited life expectancy, many old people with cancer die from unrelated causes.
2. Reduced pain sensation and a diminished inflammatory response may allow a tumour to reach a later stage in its development and to spread to other areas before it causes symptoms and is diagnosed.
3. Some cancers present in bizarre and unexpected ways.
4. Some tumours may grow more slowly in old age.

The early diagnosis of cancer in old people is difficult, but, as it is common, it always should be considered when elderly people are "failing to thrive" (Chapter 6), for it is now recognised that many patients respond well to aggressive treatment of their cancer. This should always be considered, for "cure" or at least remission is always better than "care", but the cost in terms of comparative discomfort should be assessed and discussed with the patient.

Breast Cancer

Growth of the tumour is often quite slow in old age. Needle biopsy and mammography can confirm the diagnosis. Simple surgery (lumpectomy or mastectomy) is indicated in most patients, followed by tamoxifen 20–40 mg daily. Radiotherapy has little part to play. Patients with systemic metastases often present with bony deposits and fractures. If these are in weight bearing joints, such as neck or shaft of femur, surgical treatment with internal fixation will be needed. Others may require irradiation or treatment of associated hypercalcaemia (*see section on relief of symptoms, above*). Tamoxifen should be prescribed in all cases with metastases.

Intracranial Tumours

The average annual incidence rate per 100 000 of population increases exponentially after the age of 50 years, rising from about 20 to 90/1000 000/annum by the age of 80 years. About 75% of these are malignant, being secondary metastases or gliomas. Most of the remainder are benign being mainly meningioma. The diagnosis is often difficult as the presentation mimics "stroke" with focal signs (Chapter 8), dementia (Chapter 9) or epilepsy (Chapter 8). The history should arouse suspicion as the progress of the condition will be unusual. Diagnosis of a space occupying lesion can be confirmed by an abnormal CT scan and the type confirmed by biopsy, for only then can definitive treatment be given: a meningioma requires neurosurgery, while a glioma may respond to high dosage dexamethasone. Though the response to steroids is temporary it may last for several months. When relapse occurs, dexamethasone should be stopped and the tumour allowed to take its course.

Chronic Lymphatic Leukaemia and Lymphomas

Chronic lymphatic leukaemia (CLL) is common in the old and may exist without symptoms, the first evidence of the condition being the identification of a high lymphocyte count in a routine blood test. The condition only requires treatment when the blood count exceeds 20 000/mm^3 and if recurrent infections, particularly respiratory, occur. The same comment applies to the lymphomas which can be divided into Hodgkin's lymphoma (HL) and non-Hodgkin's lymphoma (NHL). Biopsy and histological assessment of the type of lymphoma and its degree of malignancy should be attempted. Some NHLs are relatively benign and do not require treatment. The majority, particularly Hodgkin's lymphoma, will require aggressive chemotherapy. This involves the use of various cytotoxic agents in combination, as repeated courses, until remission is achieved. The oncologist or haematologist should be consulted regarding the details of treatment. While the prognosis varies with the type and staging of a lymphoma, treatment can be curative, and, failing this, often achieves a remission of up to 5 years.

Multiple Myeloma

Multiple myeloma is a proliferative disease involving marrow plasma cells, and should always be suspected when a patient has a high ESR; this is usually in excess of 100/h, but lower values may sometimes be recorded. Radiology can be misleading in old age. Fractures or collapsed vertebrae are common, but these are often accompanied by generalised bone rarefaction which disguises the focal areas of rarefaction characteristic of the disease. A high index of suspicion is necessary in this situation. The diagnosis can usually be confirmed by looking for abnormal protein bands in the plasma and by identifying the abnormal plasma cells in a marrow aspiration. Patients often show a good temporary response to chemotherapy which consists of a combination of cytotoxic agents with predisolone.

FURTHER READING

Copperman, H. (1984). *Dying at Home*. Chichester: Wiley.

Saunders, C. (1984). *The Management of Terminal Illness*. London: Edward Arnold.

Wilkes, E. (1980). *Terminal Care*. Report of the Working Group, Standing Medical Advisory Committee. DHSS: London.

Yarrick, R. and Yates, J.W. (1989). *Cancer in the Elderly*. New York: Springer.

INDEX